EAT
TO
SLEEP

What to Eat and When to Eat It
for a Good Night's Sleep—Every Night

....

KARMAN MEYER, RD, LDN

Adams Media
New York   London   Toronto   Sydney   New Delhi

A adamsmedia

Adams Media
An Imprint of Simon & Schuster, Inc.
100 Technology Center Drive
Stoughton, Massachusetts 02072

First Adams Media trade paperback edition May 2019

ADAMS MEDIA and colophon are trademarks of Simon & Schuster.

For information about special discounts for bulk purchases,
please contact Simon & Schuster Special Sales at 1-866-506-1949 or business@simonandschuster.com.

The Simon & Schuster Speakers Bureau can bring authors to your live event. For more information or to book an event contact the Simon & Schuster Speakers Bureau at 1-866-248-3049 or visit our website at www.simonspeakers.com.

Interior design by Colleen Cunningham

Manufactured in the United States of America

6 2024

Library of Congress Cataloging-in-Publication Data
Names: Meyer, Karman, author.
Title: Eat to sleep / Karman Meyer, RD, LDN.
Description: Avon, Massachusetts: Adams Media, 2019.
Includes bibliographical references.
Identifiers: LCCN 2018061010 | ISBN 9781507210284 (pb) | ISBN 9781507210291 (ebook)
Subjects: LCSH: Sleep. | Sleep disorders--Nutritional aspects. | Insomnia--Prevention. | BISAC: HEALTH & FITNESS / Sleep & Sleep Disorders. | COOKING / Health & Healing / General. | HEALTH & FITNESS / Alternative Therapies.
Classification: LCC RA786 .M49 2019 | DDC 613.7/94--dc23
LC record available at https://lccn.loc.gov/2018061010

ISBN 978-1-5072-1028-4
ISBN 978-1-5072-1029-1 (ebook)

This book is dedicated to those who are tired of feeling tired.

Contents

Introduction **7**

**Part 1
Making the Connection:
How You Sleep and
What You Eat 9**

Chapter 1
Sleep Basics and the
Food-Sleep Relationship **11**

Chapter 2
Foods That Wreak
Havoc on Sleep **27**

**Part 2
The Best Foods
for Sleep 43**

Chapter 3
Foods That Promote
Peaceful Sleep **45**

Almonds **46**
Avocados **48**
Bananas **50**
Barley **52**
Brown Rice **54**
Cantaloupe **56**
Cashews **58**
Cauliflower **60**
Celery **62**
Cereal **64**
Chamomile **66**
Cheese **68**
Chickpeas **70**
Coconut Water **72**
Cottage Cheese **74**
Cucumber **76**
Dates **78**
Edamame **80**
Eggs **82**
Figs **84**
Flaxseed **86**
Grapefruit **88**
Halibut **90**
Milk **92**
Oatmeal **94**

Orange Juice with Calcium **96**

Peppermint Tea **98**

Pistachios **100**

Prunes **102**

Pumpkin Seeds **104**

Quinoa **106**

Salmon **108**

Sardines **110**

Spinach **112**

Strawberries **114**

Sunflower Seeds **116**

Sweet Potatoes **118**

Tart Cherries **120**

Tofu **122**

Tomatoes **124**

Top Sirloin Steak **126**

Tuna **128**

Turkey **130**

Valerian Root Tea **132**

Walnuts **134**

Watermelon **136**

Whole-Grain Bread **138**

Whole-Grain Pasta **140**

Yogurt **142**

Zucchini **144**

**Part 3
A Quick-Start Plan
to Better Sleep** **147**

Chapter 4
Sleep Well Again:
Recipes and Meal Plans **149**

Chapter 5
Food and Sleep Log **187**

Appendix A
Good Sleep Checklist **191**

Appendix B
References **193**

Index **203**

Acknowledgments

There are so many people to acknowledge for making this book possible. To my family, friends, mentors, and colleagues who offered support, inspiration, and guidance over the years and during this process, thank you. I feel so fortunate to have such wonderful parents and grandparents whose support has been ever present throughout many endeavors. Thanks for fostering a desire for continual learning and growth, and being the source of my passion for cooking and love of food. To my dearest friends, thank you for believing in me and offering words of encouragement that have seen me through not only writing this book but many life events. You each mean the world to me!

Thank you to the team at Adams Media who ensured this book would be presented in its best form and for seeing the need to bring the topic of good nutrition and quality sleep into the limelight.

A special thanks to Sarah Bowers, a dietetic student at Miami University and intern, who helped analyze recipes and organize nutrition facts for this project. It's always a joy working with future dietitians and seeing what bright futures lie ahead!

Introduction

We eat to sustain life, for growth and development, for nourishment, to socialize and share meals with others, in celebration, and sometimes just for pure pleasure. But have you ever thought, "I'm going to eat this so I can sleep well tonight"? Or on the flip side of that, "I better not eat/drink this because I'll never get to sleep if I do"? What you eat and *when* you eat it can play a big role in whether a peaceful night of sleep lies ahead.

Eat to Sleep can guide you back to a better, more restful sleep through your food choices. Inside you'll find detailed descriptions of the best foods for sleep and information about how your nutritional choices impact the quality of your sleep. You'll discover how to ease your body into a better sleep using everyday foods like:

- Almonds
- Avocados
- Brown rice
- Cherries

- Oatmeal
- Salmon
- Sweet potatoes
- and so many more!

You'll also find action plans and a Food and Sleep Log to help you choose what changes will work best with your lifestyle. There's no one "best plan" that will work for everyone, but there are plenty of practical tips and strategies included in these pages that can be incorporated into almost anyone's daily routine. There are also twenty-five recipes to get you started on eating for better sleep!

This book will not only help you return to consistently great sleep and restore your natural circadian rhythm; it will also give you an appreciation for and deeper knowledge of how and why food impacts the sleep cycle. So if you're ready to see how healthful eating and delicious foods can get you back on track to sleeping soundly, read on!

PART 1

Making the Connection:
How You Sleep and What You Eat

CHAPTER 1

Sleep Basics and the Food-Sleep Relationship

Chances are that if you've picked up this book, you already understand the importance of a good night's sleep, have experienced what it's like to be without it, and are ready to restore yourself to a quality sleep routine. Whether you struggle with the occasional night of insomnia or have been missing out on quality sleep for years, this book will guide you back to better sleep through food. The foods you choose to eat and at what time during your day you choose to eat them greatly impacts your sleep cycle. By making sleep-wise food choices during the day—and especially in the hours before bed—you can restore your natural circadian rhythm and return to a better sleep. Because the fact is: good nutrition equals good sleep!

Sleep Basics

You spend about one-third of your life sleeping, so it's important to make the most of that time! Sleep, despite being a state where you aren't doing much moving, is a very active, restorative process. Important building and repair of tissues occurs while you're asleep, and memory consolidation happens when you get quality sleep. Memory consolidation is essential for learning new information and being able to recall it when awake.

It's recommended that adults get 7–8 hours of sleep each night for optimal health. Short sleep duration is considered to be 7 hours or fewer in a 24-hour period, according to the Centers for Disease Control and Prevention, and currently about a third of Americans get fewer than 7 hours of sleep each night. It seems to be a cruel joke that as kids we can sleep whenever and wherever, but as we age and our days become more hectic, the struggle to fall asleep and stay asleep becomes all too common.

The Stages of Sleep

There are five stages of sleep, each categorized based on brain-wave frequencies and biological rhythms that occur. There are REM (rapid eye movement) and non-REM phases of sleep. Stages 1–3 are non-REM phases that are followed by REM stages 4–5, during which dreaming typically occurs. REM stages are usually shorter, and once they happen, the sleep cycle starts over again.

- **Stage 1:** This is the lightest stage of sleep. Brain-wave frequencies are only slightly slower than when the person is awake, and breathing is at a normal rate.
- **Stage 2:** This is a deeper level of sleep with "sawtooth" brain waves on the electroencephalogram, and the sleeping individual is more difficult to wake.
- **Stage 3:** This is a deep sleep when bone and muscle growth occur and the body repairs tissues and strengthens the immune

system. It's very difficult to wake a sleeper in this state, and when awakened during this state, the individual is very disoriented.

- **Stages 4 and 5:** These are both REM stages that occur about 90 minutes after falling asleep. Heart rate and breathing become faster. The brain is most active in these stages, and this is when dreaming happens. While the first cycle through REM stages may last only 10 minutes, later phases can last up to 60 minutes.

The amount of time spent in REM stages decreases as we age. Infants may spend half of their time asleep in REM phases, whereas adults are usually at about 20 percent.

> **There are wrist devices and apps that can be used to determine the quality of sleep you're getting at night. If you feel like you are sleeping through the night but still wake up tired in the morning and have minimal energy during the day, a monitoring device or a sleep study done by a healthcare professional may be worth considering to determine if low energy levels are related to sleep or an underlying issue.**

Tryptophan, Serotonin, and Melatonin

Tryptophan, serotonin, and melatonin are all essential for quality sleep. Tryptophan is an amino acid essential for the production of the neurotransmitter serotonin, and serotonin is needed for the production of the hormone melatonin. Let's take a look at each of them individually.

Tryptophan

Tryptophan is an essential amino acid found in foods that contain protein, such as meats, poultry, seafood, eggs, and dairy foods. Tryptophan cannot be manufactured by the body and must be taken in through food sources. Because tryptophan is a precursor for serotonin production in the body, studies have shown that tryptophan-deficient diets can lead to a decrease in serotonin levels. There are other important nutrients required for the body to convert tryptophan into serotonin,

Tryptophan is also available in supplement form, and clinical trials have shown it provides insomnia relief, even in those with severe cases of insomnia. In studies involving L-tryptophan to restore normal sleep, it has been found that it's usually more effective in treating sleep-onset insomnia (difficulty falling asleep initially) compared to sleep-maintenance insomnia (difficulty staying asleep or waking too early) and has a cumulative effect, meaning it should be taken for at least one week before improvements may be seen in chronic insomnia patients.

including vitamin B_6, magnesium, and niacin. Tryptophan-rich foods and general recommendations for how and when to consume them will be discussed further in Chapter 3.

Serotonin

This neurotransmitter, often thought of as the "happy chemical," contributes to many functions in the body, including producing feelings of happiness and regulating appetite, digestion, sleep, and memory. It's found in both the central nervous system, which includes the brain and spinal cord, and the peripheral nervous system, inclusive of everything outside of the brain and spinal cord. Low levels of serotonin have been linked to depression, poor memory, and negative mood, and as the precursor for melatonin production, it can also impact your sleep-wake cycle. This is an important point to consider, especially since many people who suffer from depression also experience difficulty sleeping.

Unlike tryptophan, serotonin is not naturally found in foods. Ensuring that intake of tryptophan-containing foods is adequate can help keep serotonin levels in check, but you can also increase serotonin through exercise and light therapy.

Melatonin

Melatonin is a natural hormone found in the body that regulates sleep-wake cycles. When night settles in and the eyes begin perceiving darkness, melatonin is released to prepare the body for sleep. Once light appears in the morning, melatonin production decreases to help the body wake up and start the day. Studies have shown that nocturnal levels of melatonin and sleep quality start to decline at puberty, and as we move into elderly ages, sleep periods become much shorter.

If your body isn't producing enough melatonin on its own, possibly due to a lack of serotonin, you can take it synthetically in pill or liquid form. Melatonin supplements can be a great solution for adjusting sleep-wake cycles from jet lag or sleep distur- bances and for people who are blind and need assistance establishing a regular sleep pattern. Before starting any new medications or sup- plements, be sure to speak with your physician first.

The good news is that melatonin can be found naturally in certain foods. Chapter 3 will explore which foods contain melatonin and tips for how to include more of them in your diet for a natural source of this sleep- regulating hormone.

How Poor Sleep Impacts Food Choices

Sleep, nutrition, and exercise have a symbiotic relationship, either working in harmony or working against one another. Poor sleep can lead to poor eating habits, and a poor diet can negatively affect your motivation to exercise. Or maybe the domino effect starts with a lack of exercise, which then causes sleep to suffer, followed by consistently poor food choices.

Think about it: When you're sleep- deprived, do you have the motivation to hit the gym after work? And when you've had only 2 solid hours of sleep the night before, are you more likely to grab a second, third, and

While a synthetic form of melatonin can be beneficial and safe for most adults when used on a short- term basis, there are side effects that can occur if it is used for an extended period of time. Headaches, sleepiness during the day, irritability, dizzi- ness, and feelings of depression are com- monly reported side effects. The amount of time that melatonin can be used without negative side effects depends primarily on the individual, but some people have been able to use it for up to two years without problems. Melatonin should not be used with seda- tive medications as it can cause increased sleepiness.

maybe fourth cup of coffee or an energy drink to get through the day? Once one area of the healthy lifestyle cycle begins to suffer, the others are sure to follow. The opposite is true too, though. Break the negative cycle by making improvements in one area, and the others are sure to follow.

There have been numerous studies that show how we are more likely to make poor food decisions when our brains and bodies are lacking sleep. With tired minds and sluggish bodies, we are more likely to make spur-of-the-moment food decisions. When we're walking around like zombies during the day, it's all too easy to resort to the convenient "quick fix" for energy like an extra-large coffee or energy drink or that less-than-nutritious fast-food meal. Over time, unhealthy eating habits such as these can lead to unintentional weight gain and chronic disease.

How Food Choices Impact Sleep

Food is responsible for fueling everything your body does during the day and even while sleeping. Quite amazing, isn't it? According to the US Department of Agriculture's 2015–2020 *Dietary Guidelines for Americans*, the most concerning under consumed nutrients for the majority of Americans are calcium, potassium, dietary fiber, and vitamin D. Three out of four of those nutrients, and the foods they are commonly found in, have an important role in getting a good night's sleep (more on this in Chapter 3).

Low blood sugar (blood glucose) levels while sleeping can lead to a stimulation in the release of adrenaline and cortisol, which promote awakening. For example, having candy or snacking on a bag of chips before bed can lead to dips in nocturnal blood glucose levels because the carbohydrates ("sugars") in them are processed quickly by the body. A better choice for a bedtime snack would be 2 cups of homemade popcorn sprinkled with Parmesan cheese since popcorn is a whole grain and source of fiber that will allow for slower absorption of glucose into the bloodstream.

Too often we are told what not to eat rather than focusing on the foods we should be enjoying more of in order to feel better. One food or meal isn't going to make or break you—it's the overall diet that is most important. It's usually not feasible to meet all of your nutrient needs each and every day, nor would it be good for your mental health to put this much focus on trying to achieve such a goal every single day! That would require too much time, energy, and attention. Instead, think of the bigger picture from week to week. A few "check-in" questions to ask yourself during the week are:

- Have I been eating enough fiber from fresh fruits and vegetables and whole grains?
- Do I need to add in some foods rich in omega-3s for heart-health benefits?
- Am I feeling energized throughout the day? If not, maybe I need to look at my balance of carbohydrates, protein, and healthy fats or limit my intake of refined sugars or caffeine.
- Did I drink enough water or eat plenty of hydrating foods over the past few days?

By choosing to focus on overall dietary habits from week to week and getting into the mindset of what you *can* eat or should enjoy more of makes eating a more positive experience, which it should be! Eating shouldn't be a stressful experience or cause anxiety.

Along the same lines, if you are feeling hungry, don't ignore those hunger cues. Find a satisfying, nourishing snack and give your body what it needs! Skipping meals when your body is sending you signals that it's hungry is not beneficial for weight loss, and you may be missing out on important nutrients that your body needs to perform at its best.

The Trouble with Poor Sleep

The lack of sleep can penetrate and negatively influence daily activities more than one may realize. Besides feeling like you can't keep your eyes open during the day, you may also experience an inability to focus, procrastinating on tasks, forgetting important events or information, lacking motivation to exercise or participate in other activities, and making poor food choices. In the more immediate term, consistently poor sleep can lead to motor vehicle crashes or job-related accidents. In the long term, sleep deprivation and fatigue invite in chronic diseases such as anxiety, depression, stroke, cardiovascular disease, and metabolic disorders. It's common for individuals who experience poor sleep quality to also report having "poor" health, according to the Sleep Health Index. It's hard to ignore the parallel upward trend of rates of deficient sleep, obesity, diabetes, and mental health issues in America. Let's take a look at each of these concerns and how many of them overlap.

Mental Health

While anxiety and stress are often the cause of sleep troubles, the lack of sleep can then exacerbate the problem. At times, it's difficult to tell which disorder developed first: the anxiety or the sleep disorder. Research has shown that individuals diagnosed with insomnia, defined clinically as difficulty falling asleep, staying asleep, waking up tired, and rising too early in the morning, are at an increased risk of developing an anxiety disorder.

We all feel sad at different times in life, but persistent feelings of hopelessness, sadness, and a disinterest in activities once enjoyed can be signs of depression. It's estimated that 20 million people in the US suffer from depression, and while the cause is often unknown, it can be properly managed through treatment. Similar to anxiety, depression can interfere with sleep, and sometimes lack of sleep may cause or make depressive symptoms worse. Insomnia is a common diagnosis among individuals suffering from depression.

Obesity and Metabolic Disorders

The amount of research and evidence linking lack of sleep to development of obesity continues to grow, and the upward trend of sleep issues worldwide has been paralleled by the increase in obesity rates. Poor sleep leads to changes in metabolic and endocrine functions, including decreased insulin sensitivity, increased levels of ghrelin (the hormone that signals hunger to the brain), decreased levels of leptin (the hormone that signals fullness to the brain), and an increase in cortisol levels at night. Let's take a look at how each of these sleep deprivation–related changes can impact the body over time.

HUNGER HORMONES

Inadequate sleep will alter hormones that regulate hunger and fullness cues. Ghrelin, commonly known as the "hunger hormone," sends signals to the brain to increase food intake and start storing fat. Leptin is the appetite suppressor and signals to the brain that there is enough energy stored in the body. These two hunger hormones are thought of as the "yin-yang" of appetite regulation, and a lack of sleep interferes with the "fullness hormone," potentially leading to overeating at meals and possible weight gain. A 2004 study from the University of Chicago Medical Center found that research subjects who only slept for 4 hours a night, two nights in a row, had an 18 percent decrease in leptin levels and a 28 percent increase in ghrelin levels.

Studies have shown that people who are obese don't respond to leptin despite having

Recent research has even shown that lack of sleep can increase the risk for Alzheimer's disease. In a study conducted by the National Institutes of Health, researchers found that beta-amyloid, a protein "waste product" that builds up in the fluid between brain neurons, was increased during sleep deprivation. The buildup of beta-amyloid has been linked to Alzheimer's disease and the formation of plaques on neurons in the brain, which inhibits neural communication. The study found that even after one night of poor sleep, beta-amyloid deposits increased by 5 percent.

higher levels—essentially, a resistance to the hormone develops as more and more leptin is needed to suppress hunger cues, similar to how insulin resistance arises for people experiencing prediabetes and elevated blood glucose levels.

During the sixteen-year Nurses' Health Study, researchers followed approximately 68,000 women, studying their weight, sleep, diet, and lifestyle habits. At the beginning of the study none of the women were classified as obese, but by the end of the study, women who reported 5 or fewer hours of sleep per night had a 15 percent higher risk of becoming obese compared to women who slept 7 hours a night.

CORTISOL LEVELS AND CARDIOVASCULAR DISEASE

People often think about dietary factors, exercise, and genetics playing a role in heart health, but sleep is also a necessity for a healthy ticker. Individuals who have consistently poor sleep are at higher risk of cardiovascular disease, regardless of weight, activity level, age, and smoking habits.

Studies have shown that a lack of quality sleep can cause an increase at night in cortisol, a stress hormone responsible for the body's fight-or-flight response. While cortisol is vital in certain scenarios when you need to be more alert, having an elevated level of cortisol when trying to drift off to sleep is counterproductive. The higher-than-normal levels of cortisol while sleeping prevent the body from entering the deeper, restorative stages of sleep in which heart rate and blood pressure are lowered. Over time, this may lead to cardiovascular issues and elevated blood pressure during the day.

INSULIN SENSITIVITY AND DIABETES

Poor insulin sensitivity, or insulin resistance, means that your cells start requiring more and more insulin from the pancreas to take in glucose from the blood. Over time, the pancreas can become exhausted from having to produce the amount of insulin needed to keep up with glucose in the blood. Once glucose starts increasing in the blood, unable to get into cells due to a lack of insulin, it's referred to as *prediabetes* or *diabetes*.

Restless, sleepless nights can cause chronic stress on the body, resulting in higher blood sugar (glucose) levels in the bloodstream. To deal with the elevated blood glucose levels, the kidneys try to remove it from the body through urination. If you find yourself waking up frequently to go to the bathroom at night, and also going frequently during the day, elevated blood sugars may be the cause. You may also be experiencing increased thirst throughout the day. Frequent urination, increased thirst, blurry vision, and fatigue are all classic symptoms of prediabetes/elevated blood glucose. The good news here is that prediabetes can be reversed if appropriate dietary and health modifications are made. Getting quality sleep at night is a part of that health equation!

Additional Ways to Find a Good Night's Sleep

In addition to making dietary changes to help tackle sleep issues, there is a variety of other practices you can put in place to find a good night's sleep. Following are a few nonfood approaches that you can implement along with your nutritional changes. What works well for one person may not be as effective for someone else in regard to sleep, but there are only positive benefits to be had by putting any of these practices into action. Each of the recommendations in this section offers a range of benefits, but one thing they all have in common is they're each a stress reducer. If stress is a primary reason you're experiencing sleepless nights, try adding at least one or two of these practices to your daily routine!

Exercise

Physical activity offers many more benefits than just getting in shape or maintaining weight. It's essential for mental health, stress management, reducing risk of many chronic diseases, adequate energy levels during the day, and getting quality sleep at night. I personally have noticed that if I don't keep up with my usual exercise routine, my sleep begins to suffer. That alone is motivation enough for me to get back to being more physically active!

A 2011 study in the journal *Mental Health and Physical Activity* found that men and women ages eighteen through eighty-five who did 150 minutes of moderate to vigorous activity each week had a 65 percent improvement in sleep quality. They also reported feeling less tired during the day. To think of the 150 minutes per week in different terms, that's 30 minutes of moderate aerobic exercise a day, five days a week. If you're limited on time for exercise during the week, bump up the intensity of your exercise to something more vigorous and aim for 75 minutes a week.

Meditation

The word *meditation* may bring to mind images of monks living in monasteries in far-off lands, or maybe it seems like a practice that is out of reach unless you have an hour to devote to it, but meditation is something we all have access to any time of day. Meditation is simply a time to reflect or hit the pause button on your day to focus on your breath, which can be revitalizing and calming all at once. Taking the time to bring awareness to the breath can help reduce anxiety and stop racing thoughts.

Does this scenario sound familiar? You wake up an hour and a half or so before the alarm is set to go off, and rather than getting up you fight to fall back asleep to make the most of that remaining time. Lying there in bed, maybe buried under the covers, your mind starts to think about everything on the to-do list for the day and, at the same time, stressing over the fact that there's only a short period of time left before the alarm rings. This anxious state is not going to help you get back to sleep fast. Instead, if you find yourself waking up an hour or two before your alarm is set to go off, try meditating. I know this is easier said than done, but if practiced, it can be accomplished, and you can return to a peaceful sleep. I've found myself here many times before, and when I become aware of my racing thoughts, I make the conscious decision to turn off those thoughts and instead focus on my breath. In a few minutes, I'm usually back asleep until the alarm sounds. If this tactic doesn't work for you, it's best to get out of bed and go into a dimly lit room to do a quiet activity like reading a book or the newspaper or working on a crossword puzzle until you find yourself yawning and feeling sleepy again.

Writing and Journaling

When my to-do list is racing through my mind at night, I grab my notepad and jot the thoughts down. It might seem like this would only make things more stressful, seeing everything written out in front of me, but I find it helpful in moving past the racing thoughts and tabling them for the next day. It feels better to have them written down so I'm not worried all night about forgetting something! I'm able to get a night of quality sleep and then wake up refreshed, ready to tackle that list from the night before.

> **There are a number of apps available that can remind you during the day or close to bedtime to take a moment for meditation, and they even guide you through the practice. This is a great nightly routine to implement to calm the mind and clear your head before hitting the pillow.**

Maybe you just need to write down thoughts and feelings about the day in a journal to let your mind relax before bed. Journaling can be a powerful tool, and it's a great way to reflect on the positive things that may have taken place during the day.

You can use the sleep journal at the end of this book as a way to practice this relaxation technique. Journaling should be a therapeutic process, though, so if you find that keeping close track of your sleep behaviors is more detrimental than beneficial, do something different that works for you!

Reading Before Bed

Snuggling up in bed with a book is a relaxing way to end the day. It allows your mind a chance to escape from everything else that may

As a chemical compound found in the cannabis plant, cannabidiol—or CBD—has been used medicinally for centuries as a sleep aid, pain and anxiety reliever, and nausea reducer. CBD is different from the chemical compound many of us associate with marijuana, tetrahydrocannabinol (THC). Unlike THC, CBD does not provide a "high" but rather offers calming effects, so there's no reason to be concerned with feelings of paranoia or a racing heartbeat with a safe dose of CBD products. Cannabidiol is legal to purchase no matter where you live and is typically available in tinctures, pill form, and sprays. As with all new supplements or medications, you should consult your physician first. Also, be sure to purchase any CBD products from a reliable source.

have taken place and to enter a different world, if even for a few minutes.

If you are at all like me, reading in bed is a surefire way to fall asleep fast! A friend of mine recently told me she likes listening to audiobooks while drifting off to sleep. She admits she doesn't usually recall much of what happened in the book, so she's often starting in the same spot over and over, but it's an effective tool to help her fall asleep fast.

If you choose to read a book on a device in bed, be sure to use the blue light filters to avoid interfering with the body's natural circadian rhythm; otherwise, you may be counteracting the potential benefits.

Aromatherapy

Aromatherapy is the practice of using aromatic plant extracts for therapeutic purposes. The calming scent of lavender is a commonly used scent in aromatherapy, and whether you choose to use lavender essential oil, lotion, linen spray, or a lavender-infused bath soak, the plant's soothing fragrance can help you get more Zzzs. This floral species has been used since medieval periods for medicinal purposes as a sedative, as an antidepressant, and to reduce anxiety.

Essential oil diffusers have become very popular over the past few years and are great to use at night to create a calm, spa-like environment in the bedroom. Add a couple drops of lavender essential oil to a diffuser before climbing into bed and allow your mind and body to relax. Roman chamomile and neroli oil are two other essential oils that have been used along with lavender in aromatherapy for their calming qualities.

Implementing a relaxing nightly routine that includes aromatherapy helps the body and mind get accustomed to what they should be doing at that time—winding down in preparation for shut-eye!

Set Realistic Goals

Sleeping like a baby every single night probably isn't realistic—heck, even babies wake up in the middle of the night for a variety of reasons. A more realistic and attainable expectation is that most nights of the week, you should be able to get a quality 6–8 hours of sleep, with the occasional night of less than ideal sleep. Because that's life, right? It's normal that you might turn over in the middle of the night in a semi-awake state, but if you find yourself consistently unable to get back to sleep after lying awake for 20 minutes, it's time to make some changes. This book will help you to see how food choices may be interfering with your shut-eye, but it's also helpful to keep the previous nonfood approaches in mind as well as you set out on your path toward peaceful sleep.

CHAPTER 2

Foods That Wreak Havoc on Sleep

The next chapter of this book will look at how certain foods and beverages can promote peaceful sleep, but on the flip side, there are a few foods and beverages that can cause major sleep disturbances, shorting you on quality sleep. It's important to keep in mind that you don't have to immediately quit these items cold turkey—you can either reduce or slowly remove these possible problem foods and/or beverages from your daily routine. This chapter will also give you a "How to Avoid It" tip box after each sleep-depriving item to help you begin to reduce or remove it from your diet. Making dietary changes can be challenging, but remember that these action steps, when done consistently, can lead to big results (i.e., you sleeping like a baby!).

Caffeine

Caffeine is a stimulant, meaning it doesn't actually provide your body with energy, like food can. Stimulants are a class of psychoactive drug that increases activity in the brain, including elevating alertness and awareness. If you've ever tried giving up caffeinated beverages cold turkey, you've probably experienced the side effects, such as headache, irritability, and fatigue.

The beverages listed in this section are common sources of caffeine. Some may have more caffeine than others per ounce, and you'll see a chart for comparison of caffeine amounts at the end of this section.

It's important to note that caffeine affects people differently. While it can increase alertness and elevate the heart rate in some, others may not feel those side effects at all, and in fact may even feel like taking a nap after drinking a cup of coffee! Take note of how caffeine affects your body, and most importantly, if it feels like your heart rate becomes increased and you have jittery, anxious feelings, cut back on the caffeine immediately.

Coffee

This caffeinated beverage may have been your beloved friend in college when you needed to pull an all-nighter, and if you're like most people, it most likely makes a regular appearance in your daily routine, helping to get you through the day. Coffee is the number one beverage consumed worldwide, and according to a 2018 survey from the National Coffee Association USA, in America 64 percent of people consume a cup of joe on a daily basis, while 44 percent drink two to three cups.

Before you decide to completely skip over this section because you think I'm going to tell you never to drink coffee again, hear me out. I love a good cup of coffee and have certainly had days when I probably would have fallen asleep at my desk if it weren't for the jolt of caffeine from an iced coffee, so I will never be the one to say, "No more coffee!" In fact, there are some positive benefits associated with drinking coffee, including decreased risk of diabetes for life-long java drinkers. However, as with most foods and beverages, overindulging can have negative side effects, including insomnia or restless sleep.

The recommended limit for caffeine is 200 milligrams per beverage consumed at one sitting and should be limited to 400 milligrams total for one day. The timing of caffeine consumption is what is most important when considering your quality of sleep. This can vary from person to person, but drinking coffee too late in the day can interfere with a peaceful night's sleep. General recommendations are to cut off caffeine intake 8 hours before your usual bedtime. Aiming to hit the sack at 10 p.m.? Cut the caffeine off by 2 p.m. at the latest.

Beyond the stimulating effects of caffeine from coffee, the acidity of coffee could be problematic for sleep if you suffer from heartburn. Also worth considering is how much sugar is being added to your coffee. Refined sugars and their negative effects on sleep will be discussed later in this chapter.

Does this sound familiar? You wake up in the morning and have your first cup of coffee within an hour. By midmorning you're losing steam and have a second cup. After lunch, a case of the yawns and heavy eyelids hits you, so you head to the coffee maker to brew a third cup for the day. This is a caffeine crash. Rather than providing a sustained, consistent level of energy, caffeine ramps up activity in your central nervous system for a short period of time. It makes you feel more alert and energized, but once the stimulant has run its course through the body, you're left feeling sluggish.

How to Avoid It

Limit coffee intake to two (8-fluid-ounce) cups per day.

Cut off coffee consumption by 2 p.m. at the latest.

Try swapping out your afternoon cup of coffee for black tea or green tea, both of which contain half the amount or less of caffeine.

Caffeinated Teas

Maybe you're not a coffee drinker but a tea fanatic instead. While black tea can be a good stand-in when trying to cut back on your coffee intake, it still contains caffeine and should not be consumed too close to bedtime. An 8-fluid-ounce cup of black tea packs about 47 milligrams of caffeine, so if you're looking for a tea to enjoy before bed, choose an herbal tea because those are naturally caffeine-free.

A few other things to watch out for:

- Don't be fooled into thinking that chai tea is an herbal tea with no caffeine. Chai is made from black tea, so be sure to avoid drinking it late in the day or before bed.
- If you enjoy matcha tea but have a caffeine sensitivity, do not consume this grassy green tea past 2 p.m. The amount of caffeine in matcha can vary depending on the type and quality, but 1 teaspoon mixed in 12 fluid ounces of liquid will have about 70 milligrams of caffeine.

How to Avoid It

Choose herbal teas instead of black tea in the evening.

Iced tea contains the same amount of caffeine as hot, so consider swapping it for an herbal tea or water at dinnertime.

Energy Drinks

Remember how the beginning of this chapter said you don't have to give up any of these sleep-impairing foods or beverages entirely? Well, that goes completely out the window when it comes to energy drinks.

Energy drinks and energy shots have nothing good to offer your body, and they are loaded not only with caffeine but also usually with the ingredient guarana extract, which delivers twice the amount of caffeine of coffee per weight. You might argue that energy drinks do have some nutritional benefits, such as providing B vitamins, but unless you have a deficiency, which generally is not an issue for most Americans, these added vitamins are being eliminated from your body through urine and are not providing you with an energy boost.

Energy drinks can have anywhere from 27–164 milligrams of caffeine per 8-fluid-ounce serving, and 2-fluid-ounce energy shots contain 80–200 milligrams of caffeine. While one or two servings of either of these will not exceed the daily recommendation of 400 milligrams of caffeine, it's important to remember that caffeine does not provide the body with energy—it is merely a stimulant. So, if it's energy you're seeking to get you through the day, turn to nutrient-dense foods and regular exercise for consistent energy.

How to Avoid It

If at all possible (which it totally is), do your body a favor and leave energy drinks on the shelves of gas stations and grocery stores.

Swap out energy drinks for naturally caffeinated beverages since there are proven health benefits to coffee and tea.

If you're taking baby steps with this and can't give up the energy drinks just yet, set a cutoff time of 2 p.m. for drinking them.

Caffeinated Sodas

It's easy to overlook the caffeine in sodas, but if you're having issues with sleeping at night, you should take a look at how many caffeinated sodas you drink in a day. While the caffeine content of soda is less than coffee and energy drinks when compared fluid ounce to fluid ounce, the total amount of soda consumed is often much higher than coffee. The package size of soda often affects how much is consumed in one sitting. Consider how much soda you consume when you have a 12-fluid-ounce bottle, a 20-fluid-ounce bottle, or maybe a large

32-fluid-ounce beverage with a fast-food meal. Are you likely to drink all the soda, no matter what size cup or container it's served in? Not only will this affect the total calories and sugar if it's regular soda, but it also affects the amount of caffeine.

Another concern with sodas is the commonly used additive phosphoric acid, which gives soda acidity and prevents bacteria and mold growth. While phosphoric acid is made from phosphorus, a mineral our bodies need and helps to form our bones and teeth, excess phosphorus can lead to issues such as osteoporosis due to an imbalance between calcium and phosphorus, and can interfere with magnesium use. Deficient magnesium levels have been linked to insomnia, anxiety, depression, joint pain, muscle cramping, and hypertension. One soda may contain up to 500 milligrams of phosphoric acid, and the current recommended daily amount of phosphorus for men and women nineteen to fifty years old is 700 milligrams per day. If you're a regular soda drinker, it's important to consider your usual daily intake and whether you may need to add in calcium-rich beverages, such as milk, during the day to balance your calcium-phosphorus consumption.

Sodas with caffeine are also a double-edged sword because of how much sugar the regular varieties contain. Simple sugars, such as granulated sugar, high-fructose corn syrup, and other refined sugars, will be covered later in this chapter since they have also been linked to sleep disturbances.

Chances are you're more likely to drink a caffeinated soda within an hour or two before bed than a cup of coffee, so it's worth reconsidering if you think caffeine may be interfering with a restful night. If you like having a bubbly beverage before bed, consider caffeine-free options. Carbonated, flavored waters with no added sugar can be a great substitute when you need a bubbly drink. Sparkling waters have also become quite popular, and there are abundant flavor options in most grocery stores.

How to Avoid It

If you're not ready to give up your soda, consider a caffeine-free version of your favorite carbonated beverage.

Cut off caffeinated sodas 2–3 hours before bed to improve your chances of a peaceful night's sleep.

Ready to ditch the caffeine in sodas but love the bubbles? Try flavored sparkling waters with no added sugar to get your carbonation fix.

Caffeine Content of Beverages

330 mg in one (16-fluid-ounce) Starbucks Grande coffee

110 mg in one (16-fluid-ounce) Starbucks Grande Java Chip Frappuccino

108 mg in one (8-fluid-ounce) cup generic brewed coffee

76 mg in one (8.5-fluid-ounce) can Red Bull

64 mg in 1-fluid-ounce espresso

47 mg in one (8-fluid-ounce) cup brewed black tea

47 mg in one (12-fluid-ounce) can Diet Coke

28 mg in one (8-fluid-ounce) cup green tea

Dark Chocolate

While dark chocolate has its nutritional benefits, like being chock-full of antioxidants, it also contains caffeine. The cacao bean from which chocolate is derived naturally has caffeine. Therefore, the higher the cacao content and the darker the chocolate, the higher the caffeine content.

Dark chocolate is generally classified as having a cacao content of 60 percent or higher. This percentage is usually displayed on the front of the package. If there is no percentage listed and the label doesn't include "dark chocolate," it's safe to assume there is less than

60 percent cacao solids. The amount of caffeine in a chocolate bar may vary based on the cacao bean type and origin. How that caffeine will impact your ability to sleep really depends more on your tolerance for caffeine and your usual caffeine consumption during the day.

If you regularly enjoy dark chocolate before bed and are unsure if it's a culprit for your sleep troubles, try skipping it for a week or two to see if your sleep improves. Chances are that if you're sensitive to caffeine from soft drinks, tea, and coffee, then having dark chocolate even 4–5 hours before bed could possibly interfere with your sleep.

How to Avoid It

If you're sensitive to caffeine, avoid having dark chocolate 4–5 hours before going to bed.

To satisfy a chocolate craving after dinner, have a piece of milk chocolate or white chocolate paired with nuts or fruit.

Enjoy dark chocolate earlier in the day, possibly as an after-lunch treat.

Caffeine Content in Chocolate (approximate values)

12 mg in 1 tablespoon cocoa powder

20 mg in 1 ounce of Ghirardelli 60 percent dark chocolate bar

6 mg in 1 ounce milk chocolate

White chocolate contains no caffeine

Alcohol

While alcohol is a depressant and can help the body to relax, it can hinder you from entering the deep stages of sleep. It's in those deep stages of sleep that your body and brain do self-restoration: not a part you want to miss out on!

You may start to feel sleepy after a drink or two, or possibly even fall asleep, but you are more likely to wake up frequently in the middle of the night. Alcohol should not be used as a sleep aid, and if you're already experiencing insomnia, it will not provide the long-term solution you need to sleep restfully. Anticipate that alcohol may start interfering with getting your sleep on a regular basis if you consume three drinks or more on any day. Alcohol can also make snoring worse, so if you or your partner snores, expect a night of interrupted sleep.

Wine with dinner or before bed is a common nightly routine for many to unwind from the day. While this may not cause any sleep disturbances for some, if you partake in this nightly activity and are struggling to get quality sleep, it may be worth taking a week or two away from this habit to see if you wake up feeling more rested. Not only will alcohol interfere with sleep in the short-term; it can also impact nutrient levels in the body over the long-term and possibly lead to deficiencies of essential vitamins and minerals. Excess alcohol intake can deplete magnesium stores in our bones and muscle, and having inadequate levels of this mineral has been linked to insomnia, anxiety, depression, hypertension, and heart arrhythmias.

Mixed drinks may be causing double trouble when it comes to getting a good night's rest, especially if they are made with caffeinated soda, energy drinks, or other beverages that contain significant amounts of sugar. The refined sugar, caffeine, and carbonation all interfere in their own ways with sleep, but even more so when combined with alcohol.

Also, it's important to note that if you are taking any sleep medications, alcohol should be avoided, as this combination can suppress your ability to breathe. Since alcohol is a respiratory depressant, meaning it makes breathing difficult, it can also worsen sleep apnea symptoms, causing you to wake up even more frequently throughout the night.

How to Avoid It

Try a relaxing, nonalcoholic beverage like herbal tea (see additional information on herbal teas in Chapter 3).

If you want a drink in the evening, enjoy it with dinner or at least 3–4 hours before heading to bed.

For every alcoholic beverage consumed, drink two glasses of water to counteract the effects and improve your chances of sleeping restfully and avoiding dehydration.

High-Fat Foods

While a fast-food bacon cheeseburger meal with fries may hit the spot in the moment, it's highly likely that you'll lose sleep later. High-fat foods and meals stimulate stomach acid production and loosen the esophageal sphincter (the entry point of the esophagus into the stomach). Essentially, this means you are more prone to heartburn after a high-fat meal, which can make getting to sleep very difficult.

The Acceptable Macronutrient Distribution Range (AMDR) for fat is 20–35 percent of total calories for adults. If you eat approximately 2,000 calories a day, that would mean 400–700 of those calories could be from fat. To put that into grams of fat, think 44–77 grams of fat per day. This recommendation can vary based on the individual, so it's best to seek personalized nutrition care from a registered dietitian who can assess your health history and health goals.

Let's say you're aiming for 65 grams of fat per day. If you have a McDonald's Bacon Smokehouse Burger with a small order of fries for dinner, that's 56 grams of fat in one meal, or 86 percent of the recommended daily value. For a lower-fat option at McDonald's, a cheeseburger with an order of kids-sized fries and a side salad with fat-free dressing would have 17 grams of fat. That's a big difference! And if it can make a difference in how you sleep at night, I'd say it's worth considering before you order.

You might be wondering how to easily determine what foods are high in fat. Generally, fried foods, cream sauces, creamy dressings, chips, pastries and doughnuts, creamy-based soups, frozen pizzas, certain cuts of meat and poultry, hot dogs and other processed meats, and ice cream are generally higher-fat foods.

This doesn't mean these foods have to be avoided indefinitely. Believe me, I'd be very upset if someone told me no more pastries! The point here is that if you're experiencing trouble sleeping related to some indigestion at night, take a look at the foods you are consuming 4–6 hours before bedtime and on a regular basis during the week. A high-fat diet can be bad not only for sleep but also for your heart and overall health.

You might be thinking, "Aren't avocados, salmon, and nuts high in fat?" It's true that these particular foods are higher in fat, but it's the healthier type of fat (think monounsaturated, polyunsaturated, and omega-3 fatty acids) that does not negatively affect total cholesterol levels, and supports brain and cell health, among many other vital functions. For example, a 5-ounce portion of wild Alaskan salmon contains about 9 grams of total fat, with 7 of those grams being mono- or polyunsaturated fats.

How to Avoid It

If you have a high-fat dinner, take a walk afterward to aid with digestion.

Try baking commonly fried foods like chicken tenders, fish, or fries.

Be mindful of portion sizes of higher-fat foods and limit overall intake to reduce risk of heart disease and other health issues.

Refined Carbohydrates and Sugar

A sweet treat before bed might be a nightly routine, but it could also be the cause of sleep disturbances. You should consider not only the amount of refined carbohydrates you eat at night but also those that you eat throughout the day. The more sugar consumed during the day, the more likely you are to wake up in the middle of the night.

What are refined carbohydrates exactly? You may be more familiar with the term *simple carbohydrates*, which includes refined sugars and refined grains. White flour, white rice, white bread, candy, pastries and baked goods, and soda are all simple carbohydrates. Generally, this type of carbohydrate is very low in fiber and may be high in added sugars. Refined grains have been stripped of the nutritious and fiber-rich bran, germ, and endosperm, leaving them with a lower fiber content and a higher glycemic index, whereas complex carbohydrates still have these parts intact and can help stabilize blood sugars when consumed. The current recommendation from the 2015–2020 *Dietary Guidelines for Americans* is that at least half of all the grains eaten during the day should be whole grains.

Highly processed sugars and simple sugars are quickly absorbed into the bloodstream, making them fast-burning sources of energy. Foods that contain refined carbohydrates often lead to a spike in blood sugar levels and insulin levels when consumed. A rush of insulin can leave you feeling hungry after eating a meal, causing overeating and possibly weight gain.

As discussed in Chapter 1, chronically high insulin levels over time can lead to poor insulin sensitivity, or insulin resistance, and cells start requiring more and more insulin from the pancreas. If this continues, the pancreas may struggle to keep up with insulin demands, and glucose levels in the bloodstream may become elevated. Insulin is then unable to get into the cells where it is needed for energy, and prediabetes or diabetes may develop.

How to Avoid It

Choose snacks with complex carbohydrates and protein, such as whole-wheat crackers and peanut butter.

To satisfy a sweet tooth before bed, try one of the snacks listed in Chapter 4.

During the day, limit sugary beverages, including sodas, juices, lemonade, energy drinks, and specialty coffee drinks and aim to make at least half of the grains you eat whole grains.

Spicy Foods

Love having a plate of spicy chicken wings while watching *Monday Night Football*? Maybe you go a little heavy on the hot sauce at dinnertime? Spicy foods, especially for those who experience acid reflux, can certainly cause an interference with sleep.

While you could reach for the antacids to help fight off imminent heartburn, they only mask the problem and are not meant to be used long-term. With continued use, these medications slowly become ineffective, meaning you'll start taking more than recommended and still will not have relief. So if you're experiencing heartburn, listen to your body and limit spicy foods to address the problem.

Just because you may need to toss out your favorite hot sauce for the sake of sleep doesn't mean all of your food has to be bland. There are plenty of great ways to flavor your food! Try using fresh or dried herbs like basil, cilantro, thyme, rosemary, and oregano. Or instead of dousing your chicken wings in hot sauce, try a homemade garlic-parmesan sauce (unless garlic is a trigger food for your reflux) or a honey-soy sauce glaze.

How to Avoid It

Avoid eating spicy foods, especially 4–6 hours before bedtime.

Add flavor to foods with herbs and ingredients that are not spicy.

If you're experiencing reflux, try drinking a cup of ginger tea or chamomile tea to help ease digestive issues.

Acidic Foods

Nearly 60 million Americans report having heartburn at least once a month, and sometimes it can be difficult pinpointing the exact cause without some trial and error. Acidic foods may be the culprit of your acid reflux. Whether it's eating the fruit itself or drinking the juice, citrus fruit contains a lot of acid naturally, so when the stomach tries to digest it, there can be an acid overload, causing it to back up into your esophagus. The same reaction can occur with tomato-based sauces on pasta or pizza and even sliced tomatoes. Having citrus or tomatoes on an empty stomach can make symptoms even worse.

Heartburn can last a few minutes to several hours, and the longer it goes untreated, the worse it can get. As mentioned in the previous section, acid reflux is not something you want to mask by chewing a bunch of antacids. It's important to uncover what the cause of the reflux is and limit the food, as chronic reflux can lead to more serious complications.

How to Avoid It

Avoid tomato-based sauces, citrus foods, and any other acidic trigger foods 4–6 hours before going to bed.

Try low-acid varieties of orange juice if you don't want to give it up entirely, and do not drink it on an empty stomach.

If you're experiencing reflux, try drinking a cup of ginger tea or chamomile tea to help ease digestive issues.

Big Meals

As Americans, we tend to eat the most calories and largest amounts of food as our dinner meal. In many other cultures lunch is the biggest meal of the day, and dinner is something lighter. Spanish and Mediterranean cultures are good examples of this, as they enjoy small-portion meals later in the day.

As a nation, we also eat too fast. We tend to overconsume before the feeling of being stuffed and miserable hits us. To avoid the feeling of being overstuffed, try not to rush through meals. For optimal digestion and to prevent overeating, it's recommended that you take 20 minutes to eat an entire meal. Why? That's about how much time it takes for the brain to send a signal of feeling full.

It may take some practice to slow down at meals, but it's worth the effort, as several studies have shown a connection between being overweight or obese and eating too quickly. To prevent gobbling up a meal, start by limiting distractions while eating like scrolling through *Facebook* during lunch break or watching TV at dinner. Take the time to enjoy your meal and the people you might be enjoying it with. Of course, you may not have this luxury at every meal, but if you can practice this at one meal each day, it's a step in the right direction.

How to Avoid It

When dining out, if the portions served are much larger than necessary, don't stuff yourself! Get a to-go box when the food comes out and put half away immediately so you're not tempted to keep eating.

If you're at a party, don't congregate around the food table for a long period of time. Step away from the food so you're less tempted to grab "just one more." It's easy to start mindlessly eating the snack mix, even when you're no longer hungry, if you're standing next to it.

Use ChooseMyPlate.gov as a resource to help determine appropriate portion sizes of different foods.

Challenge yourself to take 20 minutes to enjoy at least one meal a day.

Dehydration

Adequate hydration is as important for quality sleep as it is for how you feel and function during the day. Dehydration can cause irritability and confusion while you're awake, but at night it can increase sleep-disruptive snoring due to dry mouth and nasal passages. It's also likely to lead to muscle cramping that jolts you awake in the middle of the night from electrolyte imbalances. In addition, if you're a mouth breather or chronic snorer or if you have sleep apnea, you're at even more risk of becoming dehydrated at night due to fluid loss.

Many people are familiar with the age-old recommendation of drinking 64 ounces of non-caffeinated fluids each day, equivalent to eight (8-ounce) glasses. Unfortunately, that recommendation falls short of how much fluid you should be consuming during the day. Women should aim for 90 fluid ounces, and men should have closer to 125 fluid ounces from beverages and food. It's best to spread out beverages and hydrating foods throughout the day rather than trying to guzzle down a liter of water before bed. Then you'll be up at night for an entirely different reason!

Dehydration is often mistaken for hunger, so if you feel like you're always hungry in between meals, make sure you are getting enough fluids. It may be that after drinking a glass of water or unsweetened tea, the feeling of hunger goes away entirely.

On average, most people meet 20 percent of their hydration needs through foods. Increasing your intake of fruits and vegetables high in water can be an easier way to meet fluid needs rather than trying to drink more non-caffeinated liquids during the day. Also, avoiding high-sodium foods like soy sauce, frozen meals, smoked and processed meats, deli meats, canned soups, chips, salted nuts, processed foods, and some cheeses can also help prevent dehydration. In the next chapter, you'll find several hydrating food choices to keep you hydrated throughout the day and night.

How to Avoid It

Enjoy hydrating foods such as cucumber, grapefruit, and watermelon, and non-caffeinated beverages like infused water or herbal tea, throughout the day.

Minimize high-sodium foods to reduce sleep issues among many other potential health problems.

Keep a reusable water bottle with you at work and while traveling to prevent getting dehydrated.

The Best Foods for Sleep

CHAPTER 3

Foods That Promote Peaceful Sleep

Many of the foods listed in this chapter work in a variety of ways to bene-fit your body and improve the quality of sleep you get at night. A few of them are natural sources of melatonin, some provide the important amino acid to help your body produce melatonin, and others provide the essen-tial nutrients needed to help your body relax as you drift off to dreamland.

As a general rule, it's best to not go to bed on a full stomach, so while many of these foods are recommended as bedtime snack options, consuming them at least an hour or two before hitting the sack is ideal, unless noted otherwise.

In this chapter, any mention of dietary reference intakes, such as Recommended Dietary Allowances (RDA) or Adequate Intake (AI), are for women, nineteen to fifty years of age, unless otherwise noted, and are based upon the 2015–2020 *Dietary Guidelines for Americans*. The RDA of a nutrient is the average daily dietary intake amount suf-ficient to meet nutrition requirements of 97–98 percent of healthy individuals of a specific gender and in a certain stage of life. The AI value is determined when there is insufficient evidence to develop an RDA and is a level believed to ensure nutritional adequacy. Individual nutrient needs will vary among males and females in various life stages and with different health needs. To see current daily nutritional goals for differing age-sex groups, visit www.health.gov for the *Dietary Guidelines for Americans*. Before making any diet changes, consult a physician and seek individualized nutrition recommendations.

All information provided in the "Nutrition Facts" for each food was sourced from the USDA National Nutrient Database for Standard Reference.

Almonds

Sleep and Health Benefits

Almonds naturally contain the sleep-regulating hormone melatonin. This tree nut also provides the body with magnesium, which may help improve sleep quality. One ounce of almonds contains 76 milligrams of magnesium and 75 milligrams of calcium to help bring on the Zzzs. While there is currently limited research specifically about almonds and the impact they have on sleep, a study published in the *Journal of Natural Medicines* in 2016 found that rats fed 400 milligrams of almond extract slept longer and more deeply than a group that did not consume almond extract.

Almonds are known for being a source of heart-healthy fats, specifically monounsaturated fat. This type of good fat can help with weight management and improve cholesterol levels as part of an overall healthy diet. If you're trying to manage your blood sugar for diabetes or lose weight, almonds are a wonderful option for a snack as long as portions are in check! Their low glycemic index is a plus for bedtime snacking since blood sugar spikes or dips in the middle of the night can cause sleep disturbances.

How and When to Enjoy

Almonds can be included at any meal and make for an easy travel snack. Enjoy almonds whole, sliced, slivered, or chopped. If you normally go for chocolate-covered almonds, choose the cocoa-dusted almonds—which make for a great dessert option to satisfy that sweet tooth! Almonds can also be finely ground in a food processor to create a crunchy coating for seafood like salmon or cod. Whether you choose to add sliced almonds on your morning oatmeal, top a salad with slivered almonds, or snack on a handful of raw almonds in the late afternoon, this tree nut is as versatile as it is nutritious.

Enjoy 1 ounce raw, unsalted almonds as a snack in the midmorning or afternoon.

Include raw almonds in a homemade trail mix.

Top your morning oatmeal or yogurt parfait with slivered or sliced almonds for added crunch.

History

Almond trees were brought to California from Spain in the 1700s, and by the turn of the twentieth century, the industry was well established. From 1970 to 2000, California's almond yield quadrupled, and the state is now the world's largest producer of almonds. With half a million acres in the central California valleys dedicated to orchards, almonds are the state's top agricultural export. What may come as a surprise is the fact that almonds are categorized botanically as a fruit, similar to nectarines, plums, or peaches.

Nutrition Facts

Almonds have more fiber, calcium, vitamin E, riboflavin, and niacin than any other tree nut and are an excellent source of magnesium. A ¼ cup of whole raw unsalted almonds contains:

Calories	207
Fat	18 g
Protein	8 g
Sodium	0 mg
Fiber	5 g
Carbohydrates	8 g
Sugar	0 g

Avocados

Sleep and Health Benefits

Avocado has made this list for its healthy fat content and the magnesium it contains. A serving of raw California avocado provides about 15 milligrams of magnesium, or 4 percent of the recommended daily value. Magnesium is linked to decreased stress levels and fewer inflammatory issues, which can help with getting a quality night of sleep. Adequate magnesium levels can also possibly reduce occurrence of migraines and extreme cramping during menstruation. The high amount of monounsaturated fat and fiber in avocados can help you feel more satisfied at a meal or snack time, meaning that you're less likely to wake up feeling hungry in the middle of the night or overeat at any particular meal during the day. For those experiencing a roller-coaster of blood sugar levels, healthy fats like those found in avocado can help to stabilize them. A dip in blood sugar levels in the middle of the night can cause restless sleep, night sweats, and headaches, and this can occur in individuals with or without diabetes.

Avocados have been studied for their positive impacts on cardiovascular health, weight management, and type 2 diabetes. With all of the health benefits avocados have to offer, try to include them in your diet at least five times a week.

How and When to Enjoy

This heart-healthy fruit is versatile and can be incorporated at any meal or snack during the day, like in smoothies or as a topping for eggs, tacos, salads, sandwiches, grain bowls, and soup. Avocado can also be used in dessert recipes when looking for a healthier fat alternative to butter or to add creaminess to a dessert such as pudding.

When shopping for avocados, consider how soon you will be eating them. If using within the same day or even the next day, it's best to choose a fruit that has a dark green skin and has a slight give when gentle pressure is applied in

Include avocado at breakfast by making the recipe for Egg on Avocado Toast with Salsa in Chapter 4.

Top salads, grain bowls, sandwiches, or tacos with avocado.

For a savory bedtime snack, spread mashed avocado onto multigrain crackers or a rice cake.

the palm of your hand. It should not feel mushy—this indicates an overripe avocado. Ripe avocados can be stored in the refrigerator to prevent over ripening.

A fruit with lighter, brighter green skin that does not give to gentle pressure will need about four to five days to ripen and should be stored at room temperature. If you need to speed up the ripening process, place avocados in a brown paper bag with a banana.

Store cut avocado in the refrigerator in an airtight container and use within a day. To prevent browning, add a small amount of lime or lemon juice to the flesh of the fruit to slow down the browning of the avocado.

History

Originating in south-central Mexico around 5000 B.C., the avocado wasn't introduced in the United States until the mid-nineteenth century. In the early 1900s, growers in California started seeing the commercial potential for the fruit.

While many Americans may be most familiar with the Hass variety, it was one of twenty-five avocado varieties in 1950. California is now the top producer of domestic avocados, growing about 90 percent of the crop for the US. One avocado tree typically produces between sixty and 150 pieces of fruit each year!

Nutrition Facts

Avocados are technically a fruit but are often thought of as a vegetable. One serving is considered to be ⅓ of a medium avocado. In one serving of California avocado, there are:

Calories	84
Fat	8 g
Protein	1 g
Sodium	4 mg
Fiber	3 g
Carbohydrates	4 g
Sugar	0 g

Bananas

Sleep and Health Benefits

The potassium and magnesium found in bananas help with blood flow and muscle contraction and can also ease muscle cramps, all of which are important when falling asleep at night. If you've experienced muscle cramps or spasms in the middle of the night, you may have heard eating a banana can remedy them.

The other sleep-relevant nutrient found in bananas is vitamin B_6 (pyridoxine). This B vitamin is involved in more than 150 enzyme reactions in the body, including nervous and immune system function and the processing of the protein, carbohydrates, and fat that you consume. It's also involved in the production of serotonin, often thought of as the "happy neurotransmitter." A deficiency of vitamin B_6 may negatively affect your mood, possibly contributing to depression, anxiety, and increased feelings of pain, all of which can interfere with quality sleep. As if that isn't reason enough to ensure B_6 intake is adequate, this vitamin is essential in the making of the sleep-promoting hormone melatonin. A banana in the morning with breakfast means you're providing the body with the right tools to construct a night of peaceful sleep!

Bananas have more naturally occurring sugars than some other fruits, but don't let that deter you from enjoying them. The variety of vitamins, minerals, and other important nutrients you get are worth the few extra grams of natural fruit sugar. This holds true even for those who have diabetes; the fiber content of bananas and other whole fruits helps prevent blood sugar spikes and the following crash one may experience from highly refined sugar sources like soda. A banana provides about 12 percent of daily fiber needs for women under the age of fifty, and 8 percent of daily fiber for men under the age of fifty, helping promote regularity.

Start the day with a banana as an oatmeal topping or paired with a boiled egg.

Include a small banana in a pre- or post-workout smoothie.

Prone to muscle cramps at night? Have a banana with nut butter before bedtime.

How and When to Enjoy

Get an entire fruit serving by including a banana in your daily diet. Bananas are great at breakfast time or enjoyed as a snack when paired with a protein, such as nut butter, Greek yogurt, or a boiled egg. My favorite way to include bananas in my weekly diet is by making peanut butter-banana toast with a sprinkle of cinnamon on top for breakfast.

They're also perfect for adding to a pre- or post-workout smoothie to help balance and replenish electrolytes and alleviate muscle cramping. Raw bananas will provide you with more potassium per serving than banana chips, but if you prefer a snack with some crunch every once in a while, try banana chips paired with almonds or walnuts.

History

Competing with the tomato for the title of the world's most consumed fruit, about 3 million tons of bananas are consumed in America each year. Many Americans had their first taste of a banana at the World's Fair in 1876. The variety of banana that most of us know and love is the Cavendish, and this popular fruit grows best in tropical countries such as Brazil, Ecuador, the Philippines, and India. Bananas were originally found in Southeast Asia and brought to the Caribbean with the first explorers.

Nutrition Facts

This popular fruit is a good source of potassium and an excellent source of vitamin B_6. A standard serving size of a medium banana, about 7", provides:

Calories	105
Fat	0 g
Protein	1 g
Sodium	0 mg
Fiber	3 g
Carbohydrates	27 g
Sugar	14 g

Barley

Sleep and Health Benefits

Barley is a whole grain and a complex carbohydrate. A complex carbohydrate is a type of slow-burning fuel, whereas simple carbohydrates are quick-burning fuel sources. Simple carbohydrates can have their place in a healthy diet, but complex carbohydrates provide the nutrition and fiber your body needs. Some examples of complex carbohydrates are apples, bananas, beans, broccoli, and whole grains such as barley, brown rice, and oatmeal. Complex carbohydrate foods like barley are also a source of vitamin B_6, the essential nutrient that's important for melatonin and serotonin production.

Chapter 1 discussed two "hunger hormones," ghrelin and leptin. Ghrelin is the appetite-promoting hormone, and its level varies throughout the day depending on food consumption. While a lack of sleep and being obese can interfere with normal activity of the two hunger hormones, there are certain foods that can help to reduce the negative effects. Complex carbohydrates are one example because they are nutrient-dense, minimally processed, and often high in fiber, all of which help control ghrelin and leave you feeling more satisfied after a meal.

Whole-grain barley is unique in that its fiber content is found throughout each part of the grain, rather than being mostly concentrated in the outer bran layer like most other grains. Pearled barley differs from whole-grain barley and is missing some or all of the bran layer, so it is lower in fiber.

The soluble fiber in barley can help reduce cholesterol, specifically the "bad" LDL cholesterol, and control blood sugar levels. With its high protein and fiber content, barley can keep you feeling satisfied between meals, preventing overeating or excessive snacking between meals.

How and When to Enjoy

As previously mentioned, there is a difference between whole-grain

Barley works well in soups in place of pastas or rice.

Try barley as a salad topper for a chewy, slightly crunchy texture.

Use barley as the base of a grain bowl topped with roasted vegetables and grilled salmon.

and pearled barley. To get the most nutritional benefits from this grain, look for hulled barley or hull-less barley in stores to ensure it still has the bran intact.

Whole-grain barley can take almost an hour to cook, so it's best to prepare a big batch at one time and keep it refrigerated or frozen until ready to use. Use it as a side dish or in soups, salads, stir-fries, or grain-based snack bars.

History

This whole grain is the fourth most produced cereal grain crop grown in the world after wheat, rice, and corn. In ancient Egypt, barley was pictured on currency and often used in religious rituals.

Barley traveled to the North American continent with Christopher Columbus in 1494. Its primary use as a cultivated crop in early America was to make beer, and it's still used to ferment malt beer today. This whole grain can be grown in a wide range of climates, including places north of the Arctic Circle to Ethiopia. The top barley exporting countries in 2017 included Australia, France, Russia, Ukraine, and Argentina.

Nutrition Facts

Barley is not a gluten-free grain, so if you have celiac disease or a gluten intolerance, avoid eating it. A 1-cup serving of cooked barley will provide:

Calories	193
Fat	1 g
Protein	4 g
Sodium	5 mg
Fiber	6 g
Carbohydrates	44 g
Sugar	0 g

Brown Rice

Sleep and Health Benefits

Brown rice, also referred to as *whole-grain rice*, differs from white rice in that it still contains the bran layer and cereal germ, making it a whole grain. Since the bran layer is still in place, brown rice contains more fiber than white rice. Naturally gluten-free, brown rice is a great grain option for those who have celiac disease or a gluten intolerance.

Brown rice is another example of a complex carbohydrate, offering numerous benefits related to getting a night of quality sleep. It's a satiating grain, so you'll end up feeling much fuller from a ½-cup serving of brown rice than you would from the same amount of white rice, plus you'll reap many more nutritional benefits from the brown rice!

Brown rice contains resistant starches, which resist digestion, meaning they do not affect blood glucose levels. Even if you don't have prediabetes or diabetes, this is good news! In addition to being a source of fiber, brown rice is beneficial for intestinal bacteria.

How and When to Enjoy

Whole-grain rice has a nuttier flavor and chewier texture than white rice and will take longer to cook than white rice, but the added nutritional benefits are worth the extra time it takes to prepare.

There are also "quick-cooking" and "instant" brown rice options available. A whole-grain option is available in most varieties of rice, such as jasmine, basmati, and short-, medium-, and long-grain. Red, black, purple, and wild rice are also whole-grain varieties.

Be mindful of portion size when enjoying grains such as rice, as it's easy to go overboard and have three to four times the recommended serving! A ½ cup of cooked rice equates to 1 ounce of grains, the suggested serving size. Of course, it's okay to eat over this recommended portion, but you'll want to take this into consideration when choosing

Swap out white rice for brown rice at home and when dining out.

Try a savory breakfast bowl made with brown rice topped with an egg and veggies.

Request brown rice for sushi rolls when available.

other grains you eat throughout the day. The amount of grains you need depends on age, sex, and intensity of exercise and activity. For more information on grains and the other food groups, refer to ChooseMyPlate.gov.

Since whole-grain rice still has the bran and germ layers attached, it's prone to spoiling quicker than white rice. To extend the shelf life, keep it stored in a dry, cool place or in the refrigerator in an airtight container.

Enjoy brown rice with stir-fries, as a savory breakfast grain topped with veggies and an egg, or in casseroles in place of white rice.

History

For thousands of years rice has been a staple crop and ingredient in Asia, and today is still an indispensable part of many diets around the world. Before the milling of rice became common practice, white rice was something only affluent families could afford, so brown rice was consumed by the majority. As the processing of grains became commonplace, the price of white rice dropped, making it affordable for the general public. Unrefined grains now have slightly higher prices than refined grains, but as people are becoming more aware of the nutrition benefits of whole grains, purchasing and consumption have increased.

Nutrition Facts

A ½-cup serving of rice is considered the appropriate portion, but generally, people eat closer to 1 cup. A 1-cup portion of cooked brown rice provides:

Calories	248
Fat	2 g
Protein	6 g
Sodium	8 mg
Fiber	3 g
Carbohydrates	52 g
Sugar	0 g

Cantaloupe

Sleep and Health Benefits

Cantaloupe is a hydrating fruit, composed of 90 percent water. As discussed in Chapter 2, adequate hydration is important for a night of restful sleep. Foods with high water content, like cantaloupe, contribute to hydration status during the day, making it easier to reach fluid recommendations.

Looking for a boost of vitamin C? Cantaloupe can help! One cup of diced cantaloupe will provide 97 percent of the daily recommended amount of vitamin C, which is important for immune health, eye health, and collagen production and maintenance. Besides providing nearly a full day's worth of vitamin C, cantaloupe is also an excellent source of vitamin A, and you'll receive a small amount of vitamin K, magnesium, folate, and vitamin B_6.

How and When to Enjoy

Although we are fortunate to have cantaloupe, along with most produce, available year-round due to imports from other countries, cantaloupes and other melons are at their peak through the summer months.

Choosing the right melon can sometimes prove difficult, but look for these important indicators: no sizable bruises, a rind that does not appear dull, and a fragrant smell. If you plan to wait a couple days before cutting your cantaloupe, buy an unripe melon and let it sit on the counter to ripen. For ripe cantaloupes, either refrigerate them until ready to use or go ahead and prepare them. Remember to wash melons before slicing into them to wash away any exterior bacteria.

To prevent the cantaloupe from absorbing odors in the refrigerator when uncut, either store it in a tightly sealed plastic bag or wrap it in plastic wrap. Keep cut melon in an airtight container in the refrigerator and use within two days.

For a classic sweet and salty combination, try cantaloupe

Rehydrate after a workout with a refreshing piece of cantaloupe.

Enjoy a side of fruit salad, including cantaloupe, at meal times.

Try blending cantaloupe into a smoothie with strawberries, banana, and Greek yogurt.

chunks wrapped in prosciutto for an easy appetizer or snack. Take this simple appetizer to the next level by sticking it on a toothpick with a cube of mozzarella cheese and fresh basil.

Enjoy a refreshing smoothie made with fresh cantaloupe, banana, strawberries, and Greek yogurt for a quick breakfast option or after a workout. Make a packed lunch a little brighter with a fresh fruit salad of cantaloupe, watermelon, grapes, blueberries, and kiwi. For a sweet summer treat, blend cantaloupe and yogurt together and create popsicles.

History

Cantaloupes are members of the Cucurbitaceae family along with cucumbers, honeydew, and watermelon, and they are commonly referred to as *muskmelons* or *Persian melons*. *Muskmelon* is actually the correct name for what we typically call *cantaloupe* in America; true cantaloupe (*Cucumis melo cantalupensis*) is grown in Europe and has a smooth skin.

In the United States, the top cantaloupe-producing states include Arizona, California, Florida, Georgia, and Texas, and this melon can be enjoyed year-round thanks to imports from Central America and Mexico during the off-season months.

Nutrition Facts

A 1-cup serving of cantaloupe cubes provides:

Calories	54
Fat	0 g
Protein	1 g
Sodium	26 mg
Fiber	1 g
Carbohydrates	13 g
Sugar	13 g

Cashews

Sleep and Health Benefits

Cashews have primarily made this list due to their magnesium content, but as with all of the foods and beverages in this chapter, they offer other nutritional benefits as well. Similar to almonds and avocado that we've already covered, cashews are a source of the mineral magnesium, which has been shown to promote quality sleep. In just a ¼-cup serving of cashews, you'll get 80 milligrams of magnesium. That's over 20 percent of the recommended daily intake!

Of all the different types of tree nuts, cashews contain the most iron, providing 1.9 milligrams in a 1-ounce portion. Iron is essential for blood production, and when iron-deficiency anemia occurs, you may feel tired and short of breath.

How and When to Enjoy

There are a number of ways to eat cashews beyond eating them whole. Cashew butter has become a popular alternative to peanut butter for those with a peanut allergy and for those who prefer the taste. Over the past few years, several vegan cashew-based products have hit the grocery store shelves, including cashew milk, cheese, cream sauces, and even mayonnaise.

Cashews make a great topping for stir-fries, Asian noodle dishes, and Indian curries. Chop them up very fine and add them to homemade energy bites or bars, or throw them into smoothies for a boost of protein, healthy fats, iron, and magnesium. You can easily make roasted, flavored cashews at home by tossing them in a small amount of oil and your favorite seasonings. Try a combination of lime zest and chili powder for a flavorful snack!

Ever heard of a cashew apple? This type of apple is to thank for the cashews we all know, but the fruit itself is only enjoyed by those who grow them or live near an orchard because they are extremely perishable.

Add cashews to a homemade trail mix along with almonds and walnuts.

Use cashews as a salad topper or on top of stir-fry dishes for crunch.

Enjoy cashews as a snack paired with fresh figs, a banana, or prunes.

History

The cashew is believed to have originated in Brazil. When Europeans first encountered them, they were thought to be inedible because the cashew is enclosed in a shell that can cause skin irritations similar to a poison ivy reaction. Native tribes showed the Europeans how to safely remove the outer shell to expose the cashew inside. It wasn't until the early 1900s that cashews made their way to the United States. Cashews are grown in warm, humid climates and have to be harvested by hand. The top cashew-producing countries across the globe include Vietnam, Nigeria, India, and Brazil.

Nutrition Facts

While cashews and other nuts offer several nutritional benefits, it can be all too easy to take more than a recommended serving size, which in terms of cashews is about 1 ounce, or 18 cashews. I recommend scooping out the appropriate portion size from a canister and then putting it away so you're less tempted to dig back in for more. By weight, cashews contain a slightly higher amount of saturated fat and carbohydrates compared to almonds and walnuts. In terms of magnesium content, though, cashews have higher levels than almonds and walnuts. A 1-ounce serving contains:

Calories	160
Fat	13 g
Protein	5 g
Sodium	110 mg
Fiber	1 g
Carbohydrates	8 g
Sugar	1 g

Cauliflower

Sleep and Health Benefits

Made up of 92 percent water, cauliflower may seem like an unassuming vegetable to choose for its nutrition value, but don't let it get by you! This cruciferous vegetable offers several nutritional benefits and has made its way on to this list of sleep-promoting foods primarily for its ability to contribute to hydration.

An additional sleep benefit of cauliflower is the potassium it contains. While it's not necessarily considered an "excellent" or even "good" source of potassium according to US Food and Drug Administration (FDA) regulations, it still contributes to the daily intake goal of 4,700 milligrams of potassium. In a 1-cup portion of chopped raw cauliflower, you'll receive 320 milligrams of potassium, nearly 7 percent of the dietary reference intake. Potassium is important for blood flow, muscle contraction, and easing muscle cramps.

Cauliflower is high in vitamin C, an important vitamin for reducing inflammation; for wound healing; for absorption of iron; and for eye, skin, and immune health.

How and When to Enjoy

Cauliflower is a versatile vegetable that can be enjoyed raw, roasted, steamed, pickled, mashed, or included in a number of recipes. If overcooked, cauliflower can have an unpleasant, sulfurous smell, so it's important to cook it briefly, or as recommended by the recipe.

You may be most familiar with white cauliflower, but there are other color varieties available, including orange, purple, brown, and green. Including one of these other color cultivars on a vegetable tray or in the weekly dinner rotation might encourage typical cauliflower skeptics to give it another try.

When choosing cauliflower, look for crisp green leaves and heads that have no discoloration. To prepare, remove the outer leaves. Cauliflower can be roasted whole or cut into florets for

Try roasted cauliflower as a different veggie to enjoy with dinner.

Swap out mashed potatoes for mashed cauliflower for a lower-carb side.

Choose raw cauliflower as a hydrating, filling snack option or add florets to a salad.

cooking. Be sure florets are similar in size so they cook at the same rate. If making riced cauliflower, place florets into a food processor to chop into small pieces, about the size of a grain of rice. This can be enjoyed either raw or cooked. Raw cauliflower should be stored in a perforated bag in the refrigerator and can last five to seven days.

There are a variety of frozen cauliflower options available that are already riced or cut into florets. These are nutritious options as well if you prefer to skip the preparation required with fresh cauliflower.

History

Cauliflower is in the same family as cabbage, broccoli, kale, and Brussels sprouts. Nearly 90 percent of the cauliflower produced in the US comes from California. This cool-season vegetable is typically harvested from October through December or December through mid-March, depending on where it is grown in California. In

2016, it was estimated that annual consumption of cauliflower was 1.7 pounds per person, according to the Agricultural Marketing Resource Center.

Nutrition Facts

The recommended daily amount of vitamin C for adults ages nineteen to fifty years old is 75–90 milligrams per day, and 1 cup of cauliflower provides 52 milligrams! In a 1-cup serving of raw chopped cauliflower you'll receive:

Calories	27
Fat	0 g
Protein	2 g
Sodium	32 mg
Fiber	2 g
Carbohydrates	5 g
Sugar	2 g

Celery

Sleep and Health Benefits

Celery is 95 percent water, making it a hydrating snack choice. Crunching on celery can help you get closer to water intake recommendations during the day. Celery has also been known to help alleviate acid reflux, most likely due to its water content helping to neutralize stomach acid. If you suffer from gastroesophageal reflux disease, try munching on a few celery sticks before turning to the antacid medications to see if you can find relief. This green veggie is also a source of potassium, important for aiding in muscle relaxation and contraction, blood flow, and easing muscle cramps.

How and When to Enjoy

Celery is usually enjoyed raw and used often in cooking and flavoring soups since it is an aromatic vegetable. When combined with apple, lemon, and cucumber, celery can be juiced to make a refreshing beverage.

To keep celery fresh, remove it from the plastic bag it may have been packed in and wrap it in aluminum foil before putting it in the refrigerator. The aluminum foil allows ethylene gas, which the celery naturally produces, to escape, helping it stay fresh longer. It's best to keep celery whole until ready to use, but if you prefer to cut celery into sticks for easy snacking, do not store them in water. Keep prepped celery sticks in an airtight container up to two days in the fridge.

Make use of celery leaves and their nutritional benefits by using them like other fresh herbs, adding them to soups or creating a homemade pesto with pine nuts and Parmesan cheese. No reason to waste a perfectly good ingredient!

History

Thought to have originated in the Mediterranean Basin, celery has been used for medicinal purposes. In ancient Ayurvedic

Pack celery as a snack along with nut butter for protein.

Use celery sticks to serve chicken salad or tuna in place of bread or crackers.

Fill celery sticks with low-fat flavored cream cheese and wrap with low-sodium deli turkey.

medicine, celery seed was used to treat colds, poor digestion, and different types of arthritis. In North America the most common type of celery is the green variety, also called *Pascal celery*. This vegetable is available year-round and is grown primarily in California and Michigan.

Calories	15
Fat	0 g
Protein	1 g
Sodium	88 mg
Fiber	2 g
Carbohydrates	3 g
Sugar	1 g

Nutrition Facts

Celery is a low-calorie food and a source of fiber. You might be surprised to see the amount of sodium in a serving of celery is about 88 milligrams. While this is higher than most fresh vegetables, celery is still a low-sodium food and can easily fit into the American Heart Association's recommendation for 1,500 milligrams of sodium a day. A typical serving of celery, about 110 grams, or six to seven (5") celery sticks, provides:

Cereal

Sleep and Health Benefits

There are endless options in the cereal aisle at the grocery store, many of which are loaded with sugar. While cereal is often fortified with vitamins and minerals, I wouldn't generally classify most of them as a nutritious breakfast option. Whole-grain cereals, however, can be better options, which will be discussed in this section.

Complex carbohydrates are beneficial in the daily diet and can improve sleep quality. When choosing breakfast cereals, look for whole-grain options since they contain more fiber than highly processed cereals. Take a look at the Nutrition Facts label for the serving size, total added sugar, and amount of dietary fiber. A general guide to selecting a healthier breakfast cereal is to find one that has 250 calories or fewer per serving, at least 5 grams of fiber per serving, and 10 grams or less of added sugar per serving.

While I don't suggest relying on a bowl of cereal and milk alone as a meal on a regular basis, if it sounds like a satisfying bedtime snack, go for it. This combination is a one-two punch when it comes to bettering sleep. The carbohydrates in the cereal and the protein in the milk work together to help keep blood sugars stabilized throughout the night, plus you'll be getting the potassium, magnesium, and phosphorus from the milk that have been shown to relieve muscle contractions.

How and When to Enjoy

Having whole-grain cereal with milk before bed is a winning combination since milk is also a sleep-promoting food. The important point to keep in mind, as always, is portion size. It's easy to pour more cereal than the recommended serving size listed on the box. To practice portion control with cereal, use the same-sized bowl each time you have it. The first few times you pour cereal from the box, use a measuring cup to see exactly what a serving size looks like in the bowl you're

Enjoy whole-grain cereal with milk as a bedtime snack.

For breakfast, have whole-grain cereal with milk and an egg for a satisfying option.

Dry cereal can be a good snack in combination with string cheese or yogurt.

using. If there's too much empty space, use a smaller bowl to make your brain think that you are getting more cereal. We eat with our eyes first, so this trick can keep you from feeling deprived. Believe me, it works! After you get used to seeing what the recommended serving size looks like in your bowl, you won't need a measuring cup anymore.

History

Breakfast cereal is an American creation, originally developed in 1863 by James Caleb Jackson. Throughout the first half of the twentieth century, several of the much-loved cereals we know today, including Corn Flakes, Wheaties, Rice Krispies, Cheerios, and Frosted Flakes, were created. During the last half of the century, breakfast cereals were formulated with more sugar and were heavily marketed toward children.

Nutrition Facts

Nutrition facts will vary among cereals, so read the nutrition label to see exactly what's in a serving. To easily find breakfast cereals that contain whole grains, look for the golden-yellow Whole Grain Stamp from the Whole Grains Council on the front of the cereal box. There are three different versions of the Whole Grain Stamp: the 100 percent stamp, the 50 percent stamp, and the basic stamp signifying that a product contains at least 8 grams of whole grains but may also contain some refined grain. Keep in mind that a cereal box may have the Whole Grain Stamp but could still be a sugar bomb, so be sure to check the nutrition label.

Chamomile

Sleep and Health Benefits

Chamomile is a plant that has been used for centuries as a sleep-inducer, to calm anxiety, and to relieve digestive issues. It's thought that the calming effects of chamomile tea occur thanks to apigenin, an antioxidant. Apigenin binds to benzodiazepine receptors in the brain to create a sedative effect, allowing the body to reach a deeper state of sleep.

In a study published in the *Journal of Advanced Nursing* in 2016, a group of eighty women who reported poor sleep quality were placed in either a control group or experimental group to evaluate how chamomile tea affected sleep quality, depression, and fatigue. The women in the experimental group drank chamomile tea for two weeks, while the control group did not. The experimental group participants had improved sleep quality, and their depression symptoms were alleviated.

This herbal tea also contains trace amounts of magnesium and potassium, two minerals important for muscle relaxation.

How and When to Enjoy

Chamomile flowers can be used in other foods and drinks, although they are much more commonly found as a tea. Chamomile tea can easily be found in most grocery stores. Some herbal teas with chamomile will also include other sleep-promoting or calming plants, such as lemon balm, valerian root, or lavender. Be sure to read the ingredient list to determine what is included in any tea you buy. Steep tea bags according to the package directions.

While chamomile has many beneficial properties, it should be avoided by certain groups of people. For example, due to lack of research and data on the effects of herbal teas on a developing fetus, it is recommended that pregnant women avoid them. While most commercial brands of herbal teas should not be an issue, it's best to talk with your doctor before

Have a cup of chamomile tea an hour before bedtime for relaxation and help with digestion.

If you have trouble staying asleep, drink chamomile tea to help you get back to sleep.

Try a linen spray that includes chamomile and use before climbing into bed at night to help you relax.

consuming herbal teas if you are pregnant. Additionally, if you have any health problems or take blood thinners, antiplatelet drugs, or NSAID painkillers regularly, consult your doctor first before drinking chamomile tea. The plant contains coumarin, which has mild blood-thinning effects.

History

As one of the oldest and most widely used medicinal herbs, chamomile is a member of the daisy family. Chamomile can be used in various forms, such as tinctures, aromatherapy, skin products, and as a tea, and has been reported to alleviate a wide array of conditions, including nausea, inflammation, and menstrual cramping. Ancient Romans recognized the healing benefits of chamomile tea and also used the flower as incense. The origin of the word *chamomile* comes from the word *chamomaela* in Greek, meaning "earth-apple" due to the apple-like scent of the flower.

Nutrition Facts

Chamomile tea is the most common way to consume this herb. As an herbal tea, it is naturally caffeine-free. Unsweetened teas are low in calories and carbohydrates, and they do not contain fat. An 8-fluid-ounce serving of unsweetened chamomile tea contains:

Calories	2
Fat	0 g
Protein	0 g
Sodium	2 mg
Fiber	0 g
Carbohydrates	0.5 g
Sugar	0 g

Cheese

Sleep and Health Benefits

Dairy foods, including cheese made from cow's milk, are a source of potassium, calcium, and magnesium, which all play a role in getting a peaceful night of sleep. Potassium and magnesium can ease muscle cramping, while calcium is important for melatonin production. Magnesium is needed by the body to transport calcium and potassium, showing just how essential this nutrient trio is for many vital functions. In addition to the sleep benefits these three nutrients offer, they also impact electrolyte balance, blood pressure, and bone health.

If you have been diagnosed with lactose intolerance or believe you're experiencing symptoms of lactose intolerance, there are cheeses that are naturally lower in lactose or lactose-free. Swiss, Cheddar, Monterey jack, and mozzarella cheese are all low-lactose options.

Cheese is also a source of protein, making it a great option to pair with a complex carbohydrate food for a snack or at a meal, and vitamin A, important for eye and skin health, immune function, growth and health of cells, and reproduction.

How and When to Enjoy

Cheese is one food that most people probably don't need suggestions for how and when to enjoy! Include cheese at a snack during the day or have it before bed paired with whole-grain crackers or a small glass of tart cherry juice. Remember to keep serving sizes in check when enjoying cheese as a snack or when using it in a recipe.

The individualized packaging of string cheese makes it easy to pack in lunch boxes for both kids and adults! String cheese can also be used to create recipes like mini English muffin pizzas, and it is great for keeping serving sizes in check since it is already wrapped in individual portions. There are plenty of other individually wrapped cheeses available in the supermarket besides string cheese that make great snack options as well.

Pack cheese as a snack along with a piece of fresh fruit.

Use low-fat cheese to top English muffin "pizzas."

Pair mozzarella string cheese with a serving of almonds, cashews, pistachios, or walnuts as a snack before bed.

History

While no one really knows who made the first cheese, it's believed that cheesemaking goes back more than 4,000 years. Italy became the center of European cheesemaking during the tenth century and continued to grow in popularity across Europe, becoming a staple of the diet. The art of cheesemaking came to America with the Pilgrims, but it wasn't until 1851 that the first cheese factory opened in the United States in New York.

Nutrition Facts

Nutrition information will vary between different types of cheese and depending on the total fat content since there are reduced-fat and fat-free varieties available. Portion size is important to keep in mind when it comes to cheese, and generally, 1 ounce is the recommended serving size. If you're watching fat in your diet, choose part-skim options like mozzarella, Swiss, Parmesan, provolone,

Cheddar, Colby, Muenster, ricotta, and cottage cheese. For lower-sodium cheese options, look for Swiss, Monterey jack, ricotta, and low-sodium varieties of Cheddar, Colby, mozzarella, and provolone. Part-skim mozzarella string cheese is a convenient cheese choice to keep on hand to have as a snack and when you need a source of protein on the go, and it is usually well accepted among both adults and kids, so you can keep everyone happy with this cheese stocked in the fridge! The following nutrition information is from a store-brand mozzarella string cheese:

Calories	80
Fat	6 g
Protein	7 g
Sodium	150 mg
Fiber	0 g
Carbohydrates	1 g
Sugar	14 g

Chickpeas

Sleep and Health Benefits

A member of the legume family, chickpeas are rich in tryptophan and contain vitamin B_6 and magnesium, which assist you in getting a restful night of sleep. Vitamin B_6, also known as *pyridoxine*, is a part of more than 150 enzyme reactions in the body, including the processing of protein, carbohydrates, and fat that you consume and proper functioning of the nervous and immune systems. Vitamin B_6 is essential for the production of serotonin, that neurotransmitter that makes us happy. When there is a deficiency of vitamin B_6, you may experience sadness or feelings of depression, anxiety, and increased feelings of pain, all of which can disrupt healthy sleep cycles. The other important role of this B vitamin? It helps make the sleep-promoting hormone melatonin. Including foods with vitamin B_6 throughout the day provides your body with the right tools it needs to sleep well at night! A 1-cup serving of chickpeas provides 1.1 milligrams of vitamin B_6.

Other health benefits of chickpeas are that they are a great source of fiber and are rich in folate for cardiovascular health. A diet high in fiber is optimal for digestive tract health and can help keep blood sugar levels in check. They also contribute to the daily potassium needs, providing about 115 milligrams in a ½-cup serving.

How and When to Enjoy

This popular legume can be enjoyed at any time of day! While chickpeas are typically included in curries, soups, stews, salads, or blended with garlic, tahini, and olive oil to make hummus, they are a versatile ingredient. They can be finely chopped and used as a base for veggie burgers, mashed along with avocado to form a protein-rich spread for toast, or blended into homemade energy bites or bars.

Garbanzo beans can be found uncooked like other beans and legumes and also canned if you

Use chickpeas in leafy green salads for added protein, fiber, and B vitamins.

Enjoy hummus with raw cucumbers, celery, carrots, and tomatoes as an afternoon snack.

Try a vegetarian chickpea stew or curry served over brown rice for dinner.

want to skip the process of cooking them. Be sure to drain and rinse canned beans before using to help reduce the sodium content by nearly 40 percent!

Now that roasted chickpeas are easy to find in the natural foods section of most grocery stores, you can pack them as a protein-rich snack to take anywhere since refrigeration isn't required. Chickpea-based hummus is another great snack choice but will need to be kept refrigerated. Serve alongside your favorite fresh veggies like cucumbers, carrots, bell pepper strips, or raw mushrooms.

History

Chickpeas and *garbanzo beans* are used interchangeably to describe the same small legume that has become very popular in the US over the past decade. This is evident by the number of hummus options in the grocery store, along with a number of other chickpea-based snacks.

This legume is native to the Mediterranean region and is commonly used in Middle Eastern, Indian, and Mediterranean dishes. In the United States, chickpeas are mainly grown in Montana, Washington, Idaho, and North Dakota, while India remains the world's largest producer, according to the Agriculture Marketing Resource Center.

Nutrition Facts

The sodium content will vary depending on whether you buy regular or low-sodium canned chickpeas. A ½-cup serving of canned garbanzo beans (chickpeas) will provide approximately:

Calories	85
Fat	2 g
Protein	5 g
Sodium	53 mg
Fiber	4 g
Carbohydrates	10 g
Sugar	0 g

Coconut Water

Sleep and Health Benefits

Coconut water is high in potassium to help alleviate muscle aches, and it's also a refreshing option for meeting your hydration goal for the day. The amount of potassium in an 8-fluid-ounce serving of coconut water may vary between different brands, but it could contain anywhere from 350–500 milligrams. In comparison, a medium banana has 422 milligrams of potassium. For both females and males ages nineteen to fifty, the adequate intake level for potassium is 4,700 milligrams a day, according to the 2015–2020 *Dietary Guidelines for Americans.*

It's important to note that while coconut water offers the benefit of providing potassium, magnesium, and sodium to help restore electrolytes in the body, it isn't a calorie-free beverage like water. Be mindful of how much coconut water you consume during the day.

How and When to Enjoy

When buying coconut water, look for one that has minimal added sugars, is unflavored, and does not come from a concentrate. While coconut water is a thirst-quenching alternative to regular water, don't make it your primary source of hydration. It's fine to enjoy postworkout or after working hard outdoors since your body needs to be replenished with electrolytes, but you still need regular H_2O.

Try infusing coconut water as you would regular water with fresh pineapple, strawberries, or watermelon. It can also be used to make homemade popsicles when blended with fresh fruit. You can also add a splash of coconut water to smoothies for a tropical taste. Remember, coconut water does not contain protein, so you'll still want to include a protein source in the smoothie, such as Greek yogurt, silken tofu, or protein powder. Try a combination of fresh pineapple, Greek yogurt, coconut water, lime juice, and mint for a

Use coconut water as a source of hydration after a workout to replenish electrolytes.

Add coconut water to smoothies as a source of liquid.

Make homemade popsicles with blended fruit and coconut water.

refreshing post-workout smoothie or breakfast option!

Coconut water can be kept at room temperature but should be refrigerated once opened. Then be sure to drink the rest of your coconut water within the recommended amount of time marked on the package.

History

Coconut water has been around for as long as the tropical fruit of coconut palms, the mighty coconut. Inside a young, green coconut you will find the coconut meat, sometimes called the *flesh*, which you typically see in grocery stores as shredded coconut flakes, along with the coconut water.

Coconuts are grown in tropical climates, and the top producers in the world include Indonesia, the Philippines, India, and Brazil. Due to the increasing popularity of coconut products over the last decade, suppliers are now struggling to keep up with current demands.

Nutrition Facts

The nutrition facts may vary based on the brand of coconut water, so be sure to read the label on the package. Following is the nutrition information for an 8-fluid-ounce serving of a popular grocery store brand of coconut water:

Calories	60
Fat	0 g
Protein	0 g
Sodium	46 mg
Fiber	0 g
Carbohydrates	15 g
Sugar	8 g

Cottage Cheese

Sleep and Health Benefits

The calcium, potassium, and magnesium in cottage cheese will aid in muscle and nerve relaxation, helping you drift off to sleep easier. These three minerals also play a role in electrolyte balance and blood pressure. Calcium is involved in melatonin production, while potassium and magnesium can minimize muscle cramping, especially important if you frequently experience disrupting muscle cramps at night that jolt you awake. Calcium and potassium rely on magnesium to be transported throughout the body, solidifying just how essential this mineral trio is for supporting various functions in the body.

Cottage cheese, like all dairy products, is a good example of a nutritious source of simple carbohydrates because it contains lactose, sometimes referred to as *milk sugar*. Lactose is a simple sugar that when digested by the body is broken down into glucose and galactose before being absorbed into the bloodstream.

There are dairy products that naturally have very minimal amounts of lactose, such as Swiss, Cheddar, and mozzarella cheeses, while some dairy products have had the lactase enzyme added to them to help people with lactose intolerance be able to digest them easier. If you have been diagnosed with lactose intolerance or believe you're experiencing the symptoms of lactose intolerance, try a lactose-free variety of cottage cheese so that you can still reap the nutritional benefits of this dairy food.

Cottage cheese has 70–125 milligrams of calcium per serving, which is much lower than the calcium per serving found in cheese like mozzarella or Cheddar at closer to 200 milligrams per serving. This is due to the draining of the whey when the cottage cheese is made. You can still count on cottage cheese to provide quality protein, potassium, magnesium, and riboflavin. Cottage cheese can be a bit higher in sodium due to the salt that's added after the

Pack an afternoon snack of cottage cheese topped with blueberries, strawberries, or other fruit.

Add cottage cheese rather than yogurt to smoothies to reduce the sugar content without sacrificing protein.

Swap out the usual yogurt parfait for a cottage cheese parfait.

curds are formed, so if you are on a reduced-sodium diet, keep portion sizes in mind or limit intake of cottage cheese.

How and When to Enjoy

There are different options of cottage cheese available at the supermarket, including small, medium, or large curds; lactose-free varieties; low-fat or fat-free options; and even an array of flavors.

Cottage cheese paired with fruit can be a satiating snack option anytime, but it's also great before bed because it provides the important combination of protein, fat, and carbohydrates to keep blood sugar levels steady throughout the night. You can also use cottage cheese as a salad topper or mixed into pasta dishes, and it works well blended into smoothies for a creaminess and a boost of protein. Try mashing it with an avocado, diced tomatoes, and garlic to create a protein-rich guacamole that you can enjoy with tortilla chips or veggies.

History

It's thought that cottage cheese may have been one of the first cheeses made in America by immigrants. This dairy food had its popularity boom in the 1950s through the early 1970s, but since then it has taken a back seat to yogurt. According to the US Department of Agriculture (USDA), the average American consumed close to 5 pounds of cottage cheese each year at the beginning of the 1970s. Now, yearly consumption of cottage cheese is closer to 2 pounds per person.

Nutrition Facts

A ½-cup serving of low-fat cottage cheese contains:

Calories	90
Fat	3 g
Protein	13 g
Sodium	450 mg
Fiber	0 g
Carbohydrates	5 g
Sugar	5 g

Cucumber

Sleep and Health Benefits

Cucumbers have the highest water content (97 percent!) of any solid food. Like cantaloupe, the high-water content of cucumbers contributes to your hydration status during the day, making it easier to reach your fluid recommendations. Cucumbers provide a source of potassium as well to help fight muscle cramping and help with water balance.

The crunchy, cool cucumber is also a melatonin-containing food. Melatonin is important for regulating your sleep-wake cycles; it has also been shown to be involved in a number of biological and physiological functions, including cardiovascular and gastrointestinal health.

Cucumbers are naturally fat-free, low in calories, and a good source of the immune-boosting nutrient vitamin C.

How and When to Enjoy

Cucumbers can be enjoyed sliced and eaten raw with hummus or vegetable dip, added to salads, or used to garnish sandwiches and wraps. For a cool summer appetizer, try blending cucumber with nonfat Greek yogurt, fresh dill, and a touch of water to make a chilled soup. While this crunchy "vegetable" is often enjoyed raw, it can also be lightly sautéed and served warm with fresh chopped dill for a unique side.

This green-skinned fruit is available in grocery stores year-round, but its peak season runs from May to August. When shopping for cucumbers, look for a dark green skin and a firm, even cylindrical shape. There shouldn't be any cuts or major soft spots on the skin. Refrigeration is best for storing cucumbers, and they should generally be used within one week. It's best to not wash whole cucumbers until ready to use. Once cut, keep cucumbers in an airtight container for up to five days.

History

Botanically speaking, the cucumber is a fruit, although we think of it

Try sliced cucumbers dipped in hummus or a Greek yogurt–based dressing for a refreshing snack option.

Top leafy green salads with diced cucumbers.

Use sliced cucumbers as a sandwich topping.

as a vegetable, and it's a member of the gourd family. It was believed to have originated in India, and when Christopher Columbus made it to Haiti in 1494, it is thought that he planted cucumbers in the region. Today, the top five cucumber-producing states in the United States are Florida, Georgia, North Carolina, Michigan, and Wisconsin, and the fruit is harvested for two main purposes: for pickling and for fresh use. Smaller cucumber varieties are often used for pickling, while the larger cucumbers, such as the hothouse variety, are often enjoyed fresh.

Calories	15
Fat	0 g
Protein	1 g
Sodium	1 mg
Fiber	1 g
Carbohydrates	2 g
Sugar	1 g

Nutrition Facts

There are different varieties of cucumbers, but they are all fairly similar in nutritional value. In a ½ cup of sliced raw cucumbers with the peel on, you'll receive:

Dates

Sleep and Health Benefits

This dried fruit may not be the prettiest looking, but it offers plenty of health benefits! When it comes to sleep, dates provide the body with vitamin B_6, the nutrient important for protein metabolism and helping convert tryptophan into serotonin.

Dates contain potassium as well, with a serving of two dates providing about 8 percent of the dietary reference intake for adult males and females ages nineteen to fifty years old. Remember that potassium plays a role in easing muscle contractions, and it also helps regulate the heartbeat and controls fluid balances, all of which can be important for getting a night of peaceful sleep.

A good source of fiber, a serving of two dates provides more than 10 percent of the recommended daily value for fiber. Dates are also naturally fat-free and low in sodium.

How and When to Enjoy

Medjool dates can satisfy any sweet tooth with their caramel-like taste. They are so intensely sweet that one or two is usually all you need to get a sweet fix. If snacking on dates by themselves isn't an appealing idea, there are many ways to use them in recipes. Try adding a couple to a smoothie along with yogurt, a banana, cardamom, cinnamon, and ground flaxseed for a delicious smoothie full of sleep-promoting nutrients. Top oatmeal and salads with chopped dates, or try a savory appetizer of cheese-stuffed dates.

Dates are available with or without the pit, so be sure you know which kind you're biting into! When buying, look for dates that are intact and do not appear dry or shriveled. Sugar crystals on the skin of the fruit is also a sign that they are past their prime. To keep dried dates fresh, store them in an airtight container in the refrigerator for up to six months.

Add a couple dates to a yogurt-based smoothie for a bit of sweet.

Try a savory appetizer of dates stuffed with cheese, such as goat cheese or blue cheese.

Include dates in your morning bowl of oatmeal for a sweet, caramel-like taste.

History

Originating in the Middle East, dates grow on date palms, which have been referred to as *trees of life* by ancient cultures. Medjool dates came to the United States for the first time from Morocco in 1927. While American date producers harvest about 33,000 tons of dates a year, Middle Eastern countries still dominate the market, producing approximately 6 million tons. One date tree can produce anywhere from 150–255 pounds of dates each year!

Nutrition Facts

There are a variety of dates, but Medjool dates are usually the easiest to find in grocery stores. Fresh dates contain about 55 percent sugar, and as they dry, the sugar becomes even more concentrated. A serving of two pitted Medjool dates contains:

Calories	133
Fat	0 g
Protein	1 g
Sodium	0 mg
Fiber	3 g
Carbohydrates	36 g
Sugar	32 g

Edamame

Sleep and Health Benefits

Edamame (pronounced eda-mom-eh) is the Japanese name for green soybeans, which are a type of legume. Soybeans contain some calcium, about 80 milligrams per ⅔-cup serving of cooked shelled edamame, and they're also a good source of potassium, providing about 10 percent of the adequate intake goal. Calcium and potassium play an important role in muscle and nerve relaxation, which can aid the body and mind in drifting off to sleep. Both of these nutrients, of course, offer a variety of other health benefits as well, such as heart health and bone health.

A 2015 published population study from Japan involving over 1,000 individuals found that those with the highest soy intake were twice as likely to sleep 7–8 hours at night, and they reported better sleep quality. The individuals in the groups that reported the highest intake of soy were consuming about two servings of soy foods, such as tofu and edamame, each day. So what did researchers find was the reason for improved sleep with consumption of soy foods?

The isoflavones, a type of plant phytoestrogen, in soybeans and soy products were found to have beneficial effects on sleep. Similar results were found in a study in Poland from 2008 involving postmenopausal women with insomnia—sleep efficiency improved in the group with increased isoflavone intake compared to the placebo group.

How and When to Enjoy

Edamame is similar in shape to the lima bean and has a slightly crunchy texture and pretty mild taste. Compared to many other soy-based foods, edamame is typically more palate-pleasing and can be a good introduction to including more soy foods in the diet.

Although traditionally enjoyed at lunch or dinner meals, there's no reason why shelled edamame couldn't be added to a savory quinoa breakfast bowl topped

Try roasted edamame as a protein-rich snack option.

Include shelled edamame in stir-fry dishes and serve over brown rice.

Order edamame as an appetizer when dining at Japanese restaurants.

with an egg for a protein-packed start to the day! Shelled edamame can also be included in soups, stir-fries, and salads, or roasted to make a crunchy snack. Unshelled edamame is what you'll find on the menu as an appetizer at most Japanese restaurants. It's important to note that the fuzzy outer pod is not edible!

Edamame can be found in the fresh produce section with the prepared vegetables, in the freezer aisle, and possibly in the snack aisle as roasted edamame. If you see the word *mukimame* on a label, that's the Japanese term for edamame that has been removed from the pod.

History

The earliest written record of the word *edamame* appeared in a note from a Japanese Buddhist in 1275, thanking an individual for the edamame he had left. It would be centuries before edamame would make an appearance in the United States. When Americans started eating more sushi in the 1980s, edamame also became more popular. More than 95 percent of the edamame consumed in the US comes from China, but domestic production of the edible green soybean is on the rise.

Nutrition Facts

Compared to other legumes, soybeans are lower in carbohydrates, and they are the only vegetable that contains all nine essential amino acids. Cooked edamame is naturally low in sodium, but pay attention to the package when buying shelled or unshelled edamame for salt that may have been added. In a $\frac{2}{3}$-cup serving of cooked shelled edamame, you'll receive approximately:

Calories	140
Fat	5 g
Protein	12 g
Sodium	5 mg
Fiber	4 g
Carbohydrates	11 g
Sugar	3 g

Eggs

Sleep and Health Benefits

Eggs offer a satisfying combination of protein and fat but also contain the essential amino acid tryptophan. As the precursor to serotonin, tryptophan is best used by the body when eaten regularly and in combination with healthy carbohydrate sources like oatmeal or whole-grain bread, perfect complements to eggs in the morning!

Another unique quality of eggs is the choline they contain inside the yolk. This essential nutrient is important for memory function, mood, and nervous system function. For pregnant women, choline is critical to help with fetal brain development and to prevent birth defects. There aren't many foods that naturally contain choline, but eggs have one of the highest amounts, with two large eggs providing more than 50 percent of the daily adequate intake goal for pregnant women and adults.

There are very few food sources of vitamin D but one egg provides 6 percent of the recommended dietary allowance. This fat-soluble vitamin is vital for developing and maintaining healthy bones, and research has shown that vitamin D can reduce the risk of chronic disease such as diabetes.

Eggs also contain lutein, which is good for your eyes and reduces the risk of macular degeneration and age-related cataracts.

Eggs often get criticized for being high in cholesterol, but recent research has shown that eating two eggs every day does not have detrimental health effects when included as part of an overall healthy diet.

Brown eggs and white eggs are equally nutritious. One large egg has thirteen essential vitamins and minerals, including vitamin D, riboflavin, choline, and vitamin A. The yolk and the egg white each contain different nutrients, so if you choose to eat one or the other, you wouldn't get the full nutrition package. About 60 percent of the protein is in the egg white, along

Boil several eggs at the beginning of the week to have along with breakfast during the workweek.

Top avocado toast with an egg for added protein.

Add a cooked egg on top of grain bowls with vegetables and beans for a filling meal.

with riboflavin and selenium, but most of the nutrients are in the yolk.

How and When to Enjoy

Eggs are a versatile and cost-effective source of quality protein. While typically thought of as a breakfast food, eggs are great at any time of day! Boiled eggs are a perfect breakfast on-the-go option paired with a piece of fresh fruit or granola bar. An over-easy egg is a delicious addition to avocado toast, roasted vegetable hash, burrito bowls, or any dish that could bene-fit from a runny yolk for extra flavor. Whether you like them sunny-side up, over hard, scrambled, boiled, or poached, eggs can be a dependable, nutritious food in the diet.

History

Most eggs in the US come from leghorn hens of the Single Comb White variety; they can lay up to 300 eggs a year. In the early twen-tieth century, eggs were primarily sourced from personal backyard

flocks or a local farmers' market. From the 1920s through the 1960s, major improvements were made to hatcheries and henhouses to reduce the spread of diseases and environmental threats, and to improve the health of the flock and egg productivity.

Nutrition Facts

All eggs are going to be similar in nutrient content unless the laying hens are fed a specific diet high in omega-3s or vitamin D. These spe-cialty diets for hens mean compa-nies can charge more for the eggs. One conventional, non-fortified large egg provides:

Calories	70
Fat	5 g
Protein	6 g
Sodium	70 mg
Fiber	0 g
Carbohydrates	0 g
Sugar	0 g

Figs

Sleep and Health Benefits

Figs contain potassium, magnesium, and calcium, which serve as muscle relaxants and can improve blood flow, easing the body so you can fall asleep effortlessly. Having adequate intake of magnesium can help reduce stress levels and inflammation in the body, important when trying to get a quality night's sleep.

Figs make a great snack anytime but are also great before bedtime to keep blood sugars stable because of their fiber content. If you usually have a sweet tooth at night, figs can help satisfy that late-night craving. Pair them with peanut butter, nuts, or a glass of milk to get a balance of slow-digesting carbohydrates, protein, and fat.

You can easily add more fiber to your diet by snacking on figs. One serving of dried figs provides 20 percent of the recommended dietary intake of fiber for women ages thirty-one to fifty. Figs also contain a small amount of vitamin A and vitamin C.

How and When to Enjoy

Fresh figs are available during the summer, while dried, canned, and frozen figs can be found year-round. When you can find fresh figs in the grocery store, they are perfect eaten as is, added to salads, sliced and used as an oatmeal or toast topping, or wrapped in thin slices of prosciutto for a sweet and salty combination. For a different take on homemade chicken salad, add fresh chopped figs.

Dried figs are a nutrient-rich snack option and pair well with peanut butter for a satisfying snack. For a filling breakfast option, spread a layer of peanut butter on toast and top with halved dried figs, hemp seeds (for some heart-healthy fats!), and a sprinkle of cinnamon.

Fresh figs should have slightly soft skin with some give, but be careful handling, as the skin can easily bruise. Ripened figs can be stored in the refrigerator, although they are best served at room temperature.

Try dried figs dipped in peanut butter for a bedtime snack.

Top leafy green salads or cooked winter squash with chopped fresh or dried figs.

Add figs to smoothies along with banana, peanut butter, and Greek yogurt.

History

Figs are thought to be the first domesticated crop, originating in southern Europe, Asia, and Africa. In the sixteenth century, figs were brought to Southern California, and that particular variety eventually became known as the *Mission fig*. Figs have been used for medicinal purposes for centuries as a diuretic and to alleviate constipation. Although figs are thought of as a fruit, they are actually a flower that has inverted into itself. The most common varieties of figs currently found in US markets are Black Mission, Brown Turkey, Kadota, and Calimyrna, with the majority being grown in California and Texas.

Nutrition Facts

In a 40-gram serving of dried Mission figs, about four pieces, you'll get:

Calories	110
Fat	0 g
Protein	1 g
Sodium	0 mg
Fiber	5 g
Carbohydrates	26 g
Sugar	20 g

Flaxseed

Sleep and Health Benefits

As a source of tryptophan and magnesium, flaxseeds offer several sleep-promoting benefits. Tryptophan may help increase serotonin levels, and magnesium plays a role in decreasing inflammation and muscle cramping. Adequate intake of magnesium has also been associated with lower levels of stress. In just 1 tablespoon of ground flaxseed, there's about 27 milligrams of magnesium.

Flaxseeds may be best known for being a source of omega-3 fatty acids, the "good" fats that we know can support heart health and brain health. Omega-3 fats also help fight inflammation in the body. Additionally, flaxseeds contain both soluble and insoluble fiber, important for reducing the risk of cardiovascular disease and diabetes and for improving gastrointestinal health.

How and When to Enjoy

Ground flaxseed is used in a variety of foods today, including crackers, oatmeal, breads, and waffles, and is emerging as an important functional food due to its many nutritional benefits. Flax oil is another way to get the benefits of flaxseeds; it can be used to make salad dressings. The great thing about ground flaxseed is that it can easily be added to foods you're already enjoying during the day, like oatmeal, yogurt, or smoothies. You can even add a serving into recipes for chili, meatballs, or pasta without changing the taste of those dishes.

Be sure to use ground flaxseed or grind whole flaxseeds before using to get the most nutritional benefits from them since whole flaxseeds are not able to be digested. An electric coffee grinder works well when you need to grind flaxseeds. If you choose to buy and grind whole flaxseeds, store them whole and only grind the amount you need when ready

For a boost of healthy fats with breakfast, include ground flaxseed in your oatmeal or yogurt.

Blend flaxseeds into smoothies to add a source of healthy fat.

Use ground flaxseed meal in baked goods to increase fiber and omega-3 fats.

to use; this will help extend the shelf life of the seeds. It's best to store ground flax in the freezer to prevent it from oxidizing or losing its nutritional quality.

When shopping for ground flaxseed, the package may say "milled" or "flax meal," but these mean the same thing. You can usually find flaxseeds or ground flax meal in the natural foods section of the grocery store or in the bulk bins.

History

Flaxseed was cultivated as early as 3000 B.C. and serves not only as a nutritional food but also as a source to create fibers for clothing (using the plant stem). The Latin name for flaxseed, *Linum usitatissimum*, means "very useful." In the 1800s, as settlers moved west throughout Canada and the northern United States, so did flax production. Canada is the world's top producer of the flaxseed plant, and generally two types of flax are

grown: flax for consumption and fiber flax for cloth-making.

Nutrition Facts

There are a couple of options available when purchasing flaxseeds, golden or brown, but the nutritional difference is minimal between them. A serving of 2 tablespoons of ground flaxseed meal provides:

Calories	70
Fat	5 g
Protein	3 g
Sodium	0 mg
Fiber	3 g
Carbohydrates	4 g
Sugar	0 g

Grapefruit

Sleep and Health Benefits

Grapefruit contains about 88 percent water, contributing significantly to your daily hydration needs, and adequate hydration during the day can impact the quality of your sleep. In addition, grapefruit is a good source of potassium. Potassium, a mineral your body requires for several functions, has been shown to have beneficial effects in both the quality of sleep and in less waking up during the night. According to the 2015–2020 *Dietary Guidelines for Americans*, most Americans are not meeting daily potassium recommendations. But with 1 cup of grapefruit sections you can get 310 milligrams of potassium. Potassium also plays a role in reducing muscle cramping, a problem that could wake you from sleep as well.

Grapefruit is also a source of magnesium and calcium, providing about 21 milligrams and 51 milligrams, respectively, in a 1-cup portion of grapefruit sections. Both of these minerals have a part in getting good sleep. If you'll recall, magnesium is involved in the transportation of calcium throughout the body, and calcium has a role in melatonin production. Adequate magnesium levels are also linked to improved mental health.

How and When to Enjoy

Grapefruit can be enjoyed raw or cooked and pairs well with creamy, healthy-fat foods like walnuts, salmon, and avocado. Canned grapefruit is also a good, nutritious option if you don't feel like cutting into a fresh grapefruit. Look for fruits canned in 100 percent fruit juice rather than syrups. Grapefruit juice is available in most grocery stores, but as with all fruit juices, it's important to watch portion sizes. Typically, a recommended serving of fruit juice is about 4–6 fluid ounces. There are more nutritional benefits to eating whole fruit than drinking the juice alone, but if it's the only way you're willing to consume it, then by all means, enjoy a serving when you'd like!

Add fresh grapefruit slices to leafy green salads or grain salads.

Use grapefruit in a fruit salsa to serve alongside grilled or baked seafood.

Enjoy grapefruit at breakfast paired with cottage cheese or yogurt.

There are several different varieties of grapefruit to choose from, including white, pink, Ruby Red, or Star Ruby. When shopping for grapefruit, look for those that feel heavy for their size and have a firm skin—there shouldn't be any noticeable soft spots. They can be kept at room temperature for a couple days, but if you plan on keeping them longer than that, wrap them in a plastic bag and keep it in the vegetable drawer of the refrigerator.

There are some concerns with grapefruit and medication interactions, so be sure to talk to your physician before adding this citrus fruit to your diet.

History

The grapefruit was first documented in 1750 in Barbados and was known as the *shaddock* until the 1800s. Brought to Florida in 1823, the grapefruit was not widely accepted upon arrival, and many citrus-lovers thought it was too sour to eat. Over the years, grapefruit has been crossed with other fruits to create the tangelo and the Minneola. In the United States, grapefruit is primarily grown in Arizona, California, Texas, and Florida and is available year-round. Per capita consumption of grapefruit went from about 24 pounds per person, including fresh and juiced, in 1978 to about 5 pounds in 2014.

Nutrition Facts

This citrus fruit is naturally fat-free, cholesterol-free, and high in vitamin C. Grapefruit is a fiber-rich fruit, making it a great option to enjoy at breakfast or for a snack. Pink and red varieties contain more vitamin A than white grapefruit. A 1-cup serving of grapefruit sections provides:

Calories	97
Fat	0 g
Protein	2 g
Sodium	0 mg
Fiber	4 g
Carbohydrates	25 g
Sugar	16 g

Halibut

Sleep and Health Benefits

Halibut is the first of several fish included in this list of sleep-promoting foods. As a source of vitamin B_6, magnesium, and the amino acid tryptophan, halibut should be included in the diet along with other seafood. Tryptophan is the body's precursor for making serotonin, the "happy" neurotransmitter, and vitamin B_6 is needed to help convert the tryptophan into serotonin. Low levels of serotonin have been linked to depression and decreased melatonin production, which can negatively impact sleep-wake cycles.

Magnesium is a key player in promoting muscle relaxation, decreasing inflammation, and lowering stress levels. These are all important factors when trying to get a night of peaceful sleep. A cooked 4-ounce halibut fillet will provide close to 10 percent of the current recommended daily allowance for magnesium.

A member of the flatfish family, halibut is also a source of omega-3 fatty acids. According to the 2015–2020 *Dietary Guidelines for Americans*, there's strong evidence showing diets that include seafood and foods rich in omega-3s are associated with reduced risk of cardiovascular disease, depression, dementia, and arthritis. A 4-ounce cooked portion of halibut provides about 400 milligrams of omega-3s.

How and When to Enjoy

This whitefish has a firm, flavorful flesh and works well in a variety of recipes. For those who typically don't enjoy fish, halibut is usually a good introduction because of its mild flavor. It can be easy to overcook, so be sure to follow recipe directions closely for appropriate cooking times based on the thickness of the halibut fillets. Using parchment paper or aluminum foil to create "pouches" for the fish while cooking in the oven or on the grill will help to keep the fish flaky and flavorful. Halibut can also be included in soups and chowders since it has a firm flesh. To help

Try oven-roasted halibut for an easy weeknight dinner option.

Feature halibut in fish tacos for a new twist on taco night.

Add halibut to a seafood chowder or tomato-based soup.

with the digestion of higher-protein meals, avoid lying down right after eating and try to eat the meals at least 3–4 hours before going to bed. A walk after lunch or dinner can aid in digestion.

Peak halibut season is late April through October, but frozen halibut is easy to find year-round. Frozen fish fillets are often an economical and convenient way to enjoy more seafood to meet the recommendation in the 2015–2020 *Dietary Guidelines for Americans* of eating seafood at least twice a week.

History

Halibut in the Atlantic Ocean was heavily overfished in the nineteenth century, so now most halibut on the market comes from the Pacific Ocean. Be aware that some halibut appears on the "Avoid" list of seafood compiled by the Monterey Bay Aquarium Seafood Watch program, due to overfishing concerns. You can visit their website (www.seafoodwatch.org) or

download their app to find out which seafood sources are recommended as "Good" or "Best" choices. The Seafood Nutrition Partnership website can also be a helpful resource when it comes to purchasing sustainable seafood (www.seafoodnutrition.org). The average halibut weighs 50–100 pounds, although one can weigh up to 1,000 pounds!

Nutrition Facts

Whether your halibut comes from the Pacific or Atlantic Ocean, it's a good source of lean protein, omega-3 fat, and vitamin B_6. A 4-ounce cooked halibut fillet provides approximately:

Calories	126
Fat	2 g
Protein	26 g
Sodium	93 mg
Fiber	0 g
Carbohydrates	0 g
Sugar	0 g

Milk

Sleep and Health Benefits

There's good reason why a cup of warm milk has been touted as a bedtime beverage around the world for generations. The nutrients in dairy foods promote muscle and nerve relaxation, which is what your body needs in order to drift off to sleep. Plus, the combination of simple carbohydrates from the milk sugar (lactose) and the protein in the milk means that blood sugar levels should remain fairly stable throughout the night, preventing any major disruptions in sleep.

Dairy foods, including cow's milk, are sources of potassium, magnesium, calcium, and vitamin D. Other health benefits of milk and dairy foods include maintaining healthy blood pressure and bone health, lowering the risk of type 2 diabetes, and aiding muscle recovery post-workout. If you believe you are lactose intolerant or if you've been diagnosed with it, there are lactose-free milks available so that you can still benefit from all of the great nutrition in this dairy food.

How and When to Enjoy

There are endless ways to use milk in recipes, but this section will focus on easy ways to drink milk during the day. Besides pouring yourself a glass of ice-cold milk to enjoy with dinner, you could also choose low-fat chocolate milk as a post-workout snack since it naturally contains the electrolytes your body needs, has 8 grams of protein, contains B vitamins for energy, and is the perfect combination of carbohydrates, protein, and fat.

I often add a small amount of milk rather than fruit juice to fruit smoothies to cut back on the total amount of sugar and to add some protein. Milk also gives the smoothie a creamier texture than adding fruit juice would provide.

Those who are not big on eating breakfast in the morning can enjoy a glass of milk or even low-fat chocolate milk instead to get

Choose 1% or 2% milk to enjoy with breakfast, lunch, or dinner.

Use milk instead of juice in smoothies for more protein and less sugar.

Try a lactose-free milk if you have been diagnosed with lactose intolerance.

the energy and nutrition the body needs after fasting throughout the night.

Of course, there's the decades-old, grandmother-tested-and-approved way of having milk—in a mug, slightly warm, and sipped before bed.

History

While milk has been consumed by humans for thousands of years, it wasn't until the fourteenth century that cow's milk became more popular than sheep's milk. The pasteurization of milk by Louis Pasteur in 1862 meant that milk became a safer product to consume and could be stored and distributed beyond the dairy farm. Wisconsin leads the way in the number of licensed dairy farms, while California, Pennsylvania, New York, and Minnesota are other top dairy-producing states.

Nutrition Facts

This section refers to cow's milk specifically and its nutrient profile.

There are a number of different options available in the milk case, from fat-free to whole-fat to lactose-free. Depending on the type of milk you prefer, the calorie and fat content will vary, but the other nutrients will be essentially the same. You'll find approximately 30 percent of the recommended daily value (DV) for calcium; 25 percent DV for phosphorus, vitamin D, and riboflavin; 11 percent DV of potassium; and 10 percent DV of vitamin A in an 8-fluid-ounce serving of 1% milk, along with:

Calories	111
Fat	3 g
Protein	8 g
Sodium	130 mg
Fiber	0 g
Carbohydrates	13 g
Sugar	12 g

Oatmeal

Sleep and Health Benefits

As a source of complex carbohydrates and magnesium, oatmeal can be a beneficial addition to your daily diet to promote peaceful sleep. One cup of cooked oatmeal contains approximately 60 milligrams of magnesium, more than 15 percent of the recommended daily allowance. This complex carbohydrate is also a source of vitamin B_6, an essential nutrient that plays a role in melatonin and serotonin production.

Complex carbohydrates, such as oatmeal, are nutrient-dense and high in fiber, which helps control ghrelin, leaving you feeling more satisfied after a meal. Oats contain beta-glucans, a type of soluble fiber that boosts the immune system and can lower blood cholesterol levels, meaning decreased risk of heart disease. The high soluble fiber content of oats plus its many other health benefits make it an ideal breakfast choice!

How and When to Enjoy

Traditionally thought of as a breakfast food, oatmeal can be incorporated into a variety of recipes or other meals throughout the day. Try using oats as a crispy coating for meats, or mixing into ground beef or turkey for burgers, meatloaf, or meatballs. A popular trend for oats now is overnight oatmeal, where oats are soaked overnight in milk to absorb the liquid and soften, then topped with the usual oatmeal toppings like cinnamon, fruit, and nuts. This is a good option in the warmer months when a bowl of hot oatmeal doesn't sound so appealing!

Oats can also be used to make homemade granola bars, granola, and energy bites, and they can be added to smoothies for a source of soluble fiber. For a healthy snack recipe that includes oats, try the Chocolate Banana Oat Bites in Chapter 4.

For convenience, buy quick-cook oatmeal or packets of plain instant oatmeal and add your own

Oatmeal is an easy breakfast option and can be customized with your favorite toppings.

Use oats to make homemade granola bars or the Chocolate Banana Oat Bites in Chapter 4.

Add 2 tablespoons–¼ cup oats to a smoothie for a boost in soluble fiber.

fresh fruit toppings, nuts, and honey for a touch of sweet. Some great oatmeal toppers that can also serve as sleep-promoters are dried tart cherries, figs, dates, strawberries, sliced banana, almonds, walnuts, and pistachios. If you prefer a savory start to the day, top oatmeal with a fried egg, sautéed mushrooms, avocado, grape tomatoes, and feta cheese for a satisfying breakfast.

Steel-cut oats have a chewier texture than rolled oats or quick-cook oats. This type of oats still contains the entire oat kernel and takes about 20–30 minutes to prepare but is often pleasing to those who thought they didn't like oatmeal because of the mushy texture.

History

Oats have a naturally sweet, nutty flavor and grow best in cooler climates that receive plenty of rainfall. The oldest cultivated oats were found in Switzerland caves, dating back to the Bronze Age.

Unlike many grains, oats rarely have their bran or germ removed when processed, meaning they remain a whole grain. Today, Russia, Canada, Finland, Poland, and the United States are the top producers of oats.

Nutrition Facts

There are a variety of instant oatmeal options out there, and then there are regular rolled oats, quick-cooking rolled oats, and steel-cut oats, so the nutrition information will vary depending on which of these you prefer. One packet (28 grams) of plain instant oatmeal, cooked with water, provides:

Calories	100
Fat	2 g
Protein	4 g
Sodium	75 mg
Fiber	3 g
Carbohydrates	19 g
Sugar	0 g

Orange Juice with Calcium

Sleep and Health Benefits

If you're not a milk drinker and don't eat enough calcium-rich foods like yogurt, cheese, bok choy, and broccoli, calcium-fortified orange juice can be a good option to get you closer to meeting your calcium goal for the day. An 8-fluid-ounce serving of calcium-fortified orange juice will provide approximately 35 percent of the recommended daily value, plus it contains vitamin D to help with calcium absorption. Calcium is important for helping the body produce the sleep-regulating hormone melatonin.

Orange juice is also a great source of potassium, the nutrient that can help fight off muscle cramping. With 450 milligrams of potassium in an 8-fluid-ounce glass, OJ can provide just as much potassium as a medium banana! You can expect a serving of orange juice to provide you with a small amount of magnesium as well, which can decrease inflammation in the body and is an important nutrient to replenish after a workout.

How and When to Enjoy

To get the most out of your orange juice, buy 100 percent juice that is fortified with calcium and vitamin D. Enjoy your glass of orange juice along with a protein food such as nuts, eggs, jerky, breakfast meat, or cheese. Just remember to keep portion sizes in check when it comes to juices!

You can find calcium-fortified orange juice in the fresh or frozen section in the grocery store. Be sure to keep orange juice refrigerated once opened or prepared from frozen concentrate, and be sure to use within five to seven days.

If you experience gastroesophageal reflux, orange juice may not be suitable if your reflux symptoms are triggered by acidic foods and beverages. There are low-acid, calcium-fortified orange juice options, but they typically contain much less calcium than other varieties.

Start the day with a small glass of orange juice with breakfast.

Blend orange juice with Greek yogurt and freeze to make home-made popsicles.

Have a small glass of OJ paired with almonds and beef jerky for a post-workout snack.

History

Before the 1920s most Americans were only familiar with eating fresh whole oranges, not drinking them. When the worldwide flu pandemic hit in 1918–1919, there was a higher awareness and demand for the immune-boosting nutrient vitamin C. Orange juice was able to provide consumers with the vitamin C they needed, and by the 1930s it became the most popular morning beverage behind coffee.

Nutrition Facts

While I typically encourage fresh fruits and veggies over juices for their fiber content, there are benefits to drinking 100 percent juices from time to time. If a glass of fortified orange juice is the surefire way to guarantee you get a healthy dose of calcium, vitamin D, potassium, and vitamin C for the day, then it can certainly fit into the daily diet. Since juices lack fiber, they are essentially a source of simple carbohydrates, meaning they will be digested quickly and

can elevate blood sugars if over-consumed or not enjoyed with a source of protein.

It's really easy to overconsume fruit juices, so be sure to pay attention to the portion size listed on the Nutrition Facts label, usually anywhere from 4 to 8 fluid ounces. A 6-fluid-ounce serving of orange juice will provide approximately:

Calories	83
Fat	0 g
Protein	1 g
Sodium	0 mg
Fiber	0 g
Carbohydrates	19 g
Sugar	17 g

Peppermint Tea

Sleep and Health Benefits

Peppermint tea offers calming, stress-reducing benefits that can help you drift off to sleep. The menthol in peppermint is a muscle relaxant, helping the body to relax and alleviate tension. If you're struggling to sleep due to sinus problems, peppermint tea and the menthol it contains can help with decongestion as well. Since peppermint tea is an herbal tea, it is naturally caffeine-free.

Peppermint tea is also known to help ease stomach upset, so if something you ate earlier in the day is bothering your tummy, try a cup of peppermint tea. If you suffer from gastroesophageal reflux disease (GERD), peppermint tea may actually make symptoms worse since it can relax the esophagus, so try a different tea, like chamomile, before bed.

Hot beverages, such as tea, help relax the body and make it easier to doze off. It's important to establish bedtime routines to train your body to prepare for sleep, and drinking a cup of hot tea is a good practice to implement. In some cases, peppermint may provide more of an energizing feeling rather than a calming one, so if you find it has the opposite effect for you, try drinking a different herbal tea at bedtime.

How and When to Enjoy

Peppermint tea is available in most grocery stores or health foods stores. If the peppermint tea contains any other ingredients, make sure that it is still a caffeine-free tea. You may find a peppermint tea blend that also includes calming ingredients such as chamomile, valerian root, or lavender. Steep tea bags according to the package directions and enjoy an hour or two before bedtime.

You can easily make peppermint tea at home using fresh mint from a garden. The amount of fresh mint you use depends on personal preference, but start with 1 cup of filtered boiling water and add about seven to eight mint

Have a cup of pep-
permint tea an hour
before bedtime.

If you're experiencing
nausea, try drinking a
cup of peppermint tea
to settle your stomach.

Pair a cup of pepper-
mint tea with cocoa-
dusted almonds for a
bedtime snack.

leaves in a tea infuser, steeping 3–5 minutes.

To store fresh peppermint leaves, lightly dampen a paper towel, then loosely wrap the mint inside. Place it inside a resealable plastic bag, sealing it with a little bit of air inside.

If you are pregnant or breast-feeding, consult your doctor about drinking peppermint tea. Also avoid peppermint tea if you are allergic to menthol.

History

Peppermint tea has been used as a natural remedy for digestive problems and muscle relaxation for thousands of years. Dried peppermint leaves have even been discovered in Egyptian pyramids.

Oregon, Washington, Idaho, Indiana, California, and Wisconsin are the top peppermint-producing states. If you'd like to have your own peppermint supply, you can easily grow this herb in small containers indoors or outdoors or in a home garden.

Nutrition Facts

Unsweetened peppermint tea is calorie-free and does not contain any carbohydrates or fat. There are only trace amounts of vitamins and minerals found in peppermint tea. An 8-fluid-ounce serving of unsweetened peppermint tea contains:

Calories	0
Fat	0 g
Protein	0 g
Sodium	0 mg
Fiber	0 g
Carbohydrates	0 g
Sugar	0 g

Pistachios

Sleep and Health Benefits

Pistachios are a good source of heart-healthy monounsaturated and polyunsaturated fats, and they have been found to contain the highest amount of melatonin, the sleep-regulating hormone, of any other nut. They also contain protein and fiber, making them a satisfying snack option, and magnesium, an important mineral for relaxing the body and helping you fall asleep and stay asleep.

If you're looking for a good source of vitamin B_6, pistachios should be on your list! In just a 1-ounce serving of roasted pistachios, you'll reach 15 percent of the recommended daily allowance of vitamin B_6 according to nutrition information provided by the American Pistachio Growers website. Remember, vitamin B_6 is important for converting tryptophan into serotonin and then melatonin. A deficiency of this B vitamin has been linked to depression and mood disorders that can lead to insomnia.

How and When to Enjoy

Pistachios, unlike many other nuts, can easily be found in stores either shelled or unshelled. Having the pistachios with their shell still intact as a snack usually means they will last a little longer and prevent you from eating too quickly!

Enjoy them on their own or paired with fresh fruit, as a crunchy topping for yogurt or oatmeal, or chopped finely to use as a coating for fish. Pistachios also work well mixed into leafy green salads or grain-based salads. If you make homemade granola bars or energy bites, pistachios are a good nut to add to these types of recipes.

Pistachio trees are wind pollinated rather than being pollinated by bees. One male tree can pollinate up to thirty female trees.

History

Pistachio trees have been in Middle Eastern countries for thousands of years and are even mentioned in the Old Testament

Keep single-serving packages of unshelled pistachios on hand as a snack.

Top oatmeal or yogurt with shelled pistachios.

Include pistachios in homemade trail mix or granola bars.

of the Bible. Despite the ancient history of pistachios, it wasn't until 1976 that the first commercial crop of the nut was produced in America. The first crop produced 1.5 million pounds, and the pistachio's popularity has been growing ever since. In 2016 a record 900 million pounds of pistachios were harvested.

California, Arizona, and New Mexico are the top states producing pistachios, and there are approximately 950 pistachio growers in the United States, according to the American Pistachio Growers.

Nutrition Facts

While the total fat content of pistachios may seem high, they are providing the body with monounsaturated and polyunsaturated fats, also known as the "good fats." Pistachios are naturally cholesterol-free. The sodium content of pistachios will depend on whether they have been salted in processing. You can expect a 1-ounce serving of salted pistachio

kernels to provide close to 120 milligrams of sodium, so if you're watching sodium intake, opt for the unsalted varieties. In a 1-ounce serving of unsalted shelled pistachios, which is about fifty pistachios, you'll receive:

Calories	159
Fat	13 g
Protein	6 g
Sodium	0 mg
Fiber	3 g
Carbohydrates	8 g
Sugar	2 g

Prunes

Sleep and Health Benefits

This dried fruit may not have the most glamorous reputation, but prunes have plenty of alluring health benefits. Most commonly associated with helping with regular bowel movements, dried plums also deliver a healthy dose of potassium. Prune juice contains 530 milligrams of potassium per ¾-cup serving—that's about 12 percent of the adequate intake recommendation for men and women ages nineteen to fifty years old.

Prunes are also a source of magnesium, providing about 16 milligrams in a serving of four prunes. Magnesium can help decrease stress levels and inflammation and may even decrease the occurrence of migraines. The potassium and magnesium in prunes not only offer sleep-promoting benefits; they also contribute to bone health. A study published in a 2011 edition of the *British Journal of Nutrition* found that postmenopausal women who ate 100 grams, or about ten prunes, a day saw an increase in bone density compared to those who did not.

Dried plums contain vitamin B_6, the nutrient that is important for converting tryptophan to serotonin. When serotonin levels are low, it is likely that melatonin levels will also be low, which can negatively affect sleep-wake cycles.

How and When to Enjoy

Prunes are available year-round and can be eaten by themselves to satisfy a sweet tooth or used in an array of sweet or savory recipes. Add chopped prunes to smoothies, homemade baked goods, grain-based salads, and oatmeal, or purée them to make sauces. The sweetness of prunes can also pair well with meats like beef, chicken, or pork. Prunes work well when you want to reduce the calories and fat in baked goods. Similar to using applesauce in baked goods in place of fat, prune purée is another healthy baking swap.

Add chopped prunes to a quinoa salad along with arugula and goat cheese.

Reduce calories and fat in some baked goods by using puréed prunes in place of butter.

Top oatmeal with chopped prunes and walnuts for a fiber-filled start to the day.

When buying prunes, look for those with a bluish-black skin that are slightly soft. Keep prunes stored in an airtight container in a cool, dry place up to six months.

Calories	91
Fat	0 g
Protein	1 g
Sodium	1 mg
Fiber	3 g
Carbohydrates	25 g
Sugar	14 g

History

With a history dating back to ancient Roman empires, prunes were a desired fruit to have during winter because they could be easily stored. While sun-drying was the original way to turn plums into prunes, today commercial dehydration has taken over the drying process. On many US packages of prunes, you will also see "dried plums," which was added to labels in 2001 in hopes of making them more appealing to consumers.

Nutrition Facts

Prunes are naturally cholesterol- and fat-free. They're a good source of fiber—part of the reason they've become known as a food good for regularity! A serving of four prunes will provide:

Pumpkin Seeds

Sleep and Health Benefits

Pumpkin seeds, also known as *pepitas*, offer sleep benefits by providing the body with healthy doses of magnesium. A 1-ounce serving of pumpkin seeds can deliver about 37 percent of the recommended daily amount for magnesium, making them one of the best food sources of the mineral. American diets are often lacking in magnesium, so snacking on pumpkin seeds is a great way to boost your daily intake! Magnesium is involved in more than 600 chemical reactions in the body and plays a key role in blood pressure, bone health, and getting a night of quality sleep.

Pumpkin seeds are also a good source of the antioxidant vitamin E, which can protect cells from free-radical damage, improve immune system function, and reduce inflammation.

How and When to Enjoy

Don't wait until you clean out a pumpkin at Halloween to enjoy the nutritious seeds inside! Available year-round, pumpkin seeds can be eaten raw or roasted, salted or unsalted, with or without a hull, and either on their own or added to recipes. If you first thought of the white-colored seeds, those are pumpkin seeds that still have the hull, while those without the hull are green in color. My favorite way to eat them is raw, without the hull, and unsalted in homemade trail mix with dried cranberries, dark chocolate chips, and almonds. They also taste great on top of butternut squash soup for a nice crunch! It's easy to add them to oatmeal or yogurt in the morning and to salads for lunch or dinner. If you're making pumpkin muffins or pumpkin bread, pumpkin seeds on top are a natural fit.

History

Native to the Americas, the oldest domesticated pumpkin seeds were found in the Oaxaca region of Mexico and are believed to be nearly 10,000 years old. The

Add pumpkin seeds to a homemade trail mix along with nuts and dried fruit.

Top oatmeal or yogurt parfaits with raw pumpkin seeds.

Sprinkle pumpkin seeds into salads or on top of soups to add some crunch.

calabaza pumpkin is a commonly found pumpkin variety in Mexican markets today, and the pepitas inside are often thrown onto the griddle (*comal*) and salted before being enjoyed. Pumpkins and their seeds have been used in a number of ways medicinally by different cultures around the world, including for diuretic purposes, prostate health, and kidney health.

Calories	170
Fat	15 g
Protein	9 g
Sodium	5 mg
Fiber	2 g
Carbohydrates	3 g
Sugar	1 g

Nutrition Facts

Pumpkin seeds offer protein and fiber, and are low in carbohydrates. While pumpkin seeds contain a significant amount of fat, they are mostly polyunsaturated and monounsaturated fats, which are good types of fat. There are salted and unsalted varieties of pumpkin seeds, so the sodium content will vary between them. A ¼-cup portion of raw, unsalted pumpkin kernels provides:

Quinoa

Sleep and Health Benefits

Quinoa (pronounced keen-wah) is a source of complex carbohydrates and provides 8 grams of protein per 1 cup (cooked). Often thought of as a grain, quinoa is technically a seed but has some similar nutrition qualities as whole grains, such as having a high fiber content, which makes it a filling and satisfying option that can help control ghrelin (the appetite-promoting hormone).

A source of magnesium, quinoa provides about 89 milligrams in a ¾ cup cooked portion. Magnesium can provide relief from muscle cramping, can decrease stress and inflammation, and may reduce the occurrence of migraines. Quinoa also contains tryptophan, the amino acid that plays a role in serotonin production.

How and When to Enjoy

This pseudograin is versatile and can be used in sweet or savory recipes. It has a slightly nutty flavor and takes on the flavors of whatever it is cooked in or seasoned with. Try swapping in quinoa for oatmeal some mornings or use it in place of rice when making stir-fry dishes. Chapter 4 includes a few quinoa recipes to try.

Quinoa is light and fluffy when cooked and usually takes less time to cook than other whole grains. There are different colors of quinoa, including white, red, purple, black, and yellow, and they can also be found in blends of the differing colors. The taste is essentially the same no matter which color you buy.

It's important to wash quinoa in a fine-mesh strainer to remove the bitter outer coating or buy the prewashed varieties. To cook, use a ratio of two parts liquid, either water or broth, to one part quinoa. You can expect 1 cup of dry quinoa to yield about 3 cups cooked.

History

Quinoa is considered an "ancient grain," having been cultivated

Go savory for break-
fast and try the recipe
for Greek Quinoa
Breakfast Bowl in
Chapter 4.

Use cooked quinoa as
a salad topping for a
source of protein and
fiber.

Serve seared salmon,
halibut, or tuna over
a bed of quinoa and
vegetables.

for nearly 5,000 years, although it has more recently grown in popularity in the United States. Native to South America, quinoa was a prominent food source for the Incas. According to the Agricultural Marketing Resource Center, there was a significant increase in quinoa consumption from 2007–2013, with imports growing from 7 million pounds to 70 million pounds.

Calories	166
Fat	2 g
Protein	6 g
Sodium	10 mg
Fiber	4 g
Carbohydrates	29 g
Sugar	1 g

Nutrition Facts

Quinoa is unique in that it contains all nine essential amino acids, making it a complete source of protein, which most plant-based proteins are not. A ¾-cup cooked portion of quinoa provides approximately:

Salmon

Sleep and Health Benefits

While you may be familiar with the heart-health benefits salmon offers, you may not think of it as a food that can positively impact sleep. Salmon is an excellent source of the serotonin- and melatonin-boosting vitamin pyridoxine (a.k.a. vitamin B_6).

Magnesium is another beneficial sleep nutrient found in salmon. This mineral contributes to the anti-inflammatory properties of salmon, along with omega-3 fatty acids, and can help reduce muscle cramping and the occurrence of migraines. In a 5-ounce portion of raw wild Alaskan salmon, there are 41 milligrams of magnesium, which is equivalent to about 12 percent of the recommended daily allowance for women ages thirty-one to fifty.

Salmon is an excellent way to get the heart-healthy, brain-benefiting omega-3 fatty acids. The National Institutes of Health recommends females ages nineteen and older get 1.1 grams of omega-3s per day and males nineteen and older, 1.6 grams per day. A 3-ounce portion of wild king salmon or farmed Atlantic salmon provides 1.2 grams of omega-3s! The 2015–2020 *Dietary Guidelines for Americans* states that there's strong evidence showing diets that include seafood and foods rich in omega-3s are associated with reduced risk of cardiovascular disease, depression, dementia, and arthritis.

How and When to Enjoy

Aim to include salmon in your weekly meal plan for its many nutritional benefits. Salmon can be cooked on the stovetop in a skillet, baked in the oven in an aluminum foil pack, made into salmon burgers, or mixed into casseroles and soups.

Whether you choose to buy fresh, canned, or frozen, you'll still be receiving the nutrition benefits salmon has to offer. Of course, fresh salmon will need to be prepared sooner than frozen or canned varieties, so be sure to

Try grilled or oven-baked salmon on top of a leafy green salad as part of your weekly meal plan.

Enjoy protein-rich smoked salmon for breakfast on a whole-wheat bagel.

Make an easy weeknight dinner like the Sheet Pan Salmon and Vegetables in Chapter 4.

use it within one to two days of purchasing. Frozen salmon should be thawed in the refrigerator overnight. Canned salmon is very convenient to keep on hand and is higher in calcium than fresh or frozen if the bones are included. Salmon bones? Yes! When salmon is canned, the canning process softens the bones, making them edible and easy to break apart, so you can safely eat them and benefit from the extra calcium. Try making salmon cakes with canned salmon and serve alongside a salad.

History

Salmon has been a staple in European diets for hundreds of years and was often smoked or cured to have as a protein source year-round. In the 1840s, New England states began canning salmon.

There are six species of Pacific salmon: sockeye, coho, chum, king or Chinook, pink, and the cherry salmon.

Nutrition Facts

The nutrition facts may vary slightly depending on where the salmon is sourced, if it's wild or farm-raised, and if it's smoked or cured. If you have specific questions about the sourcing of seafood, visit the websites for the Seafood Nutrition Partnership (www.seafood nutrition.org/) and the Monterey Bay Aquarium Seafood Watch program (www.seafoodwatch.org). You can also download an app for the latter. A 5-ounce portion of raw wild Alaskan salmon provides:

Calories	201
Fat	9 g
Protein	28 g
Sodium	62 mg
Fiber	0 g
Carbohydrates	0 g
Sugar	0 g

Sardines

Sleep and Health Benefits

This tiny fish doesn't always get the respect it deserves! One of the best nondairy sources of calcium, sardines pack a whopping 32 percent of the recommended daily value for calcium in just seven sardine fillets. Calcium, as we know, is important for helping the body make melatonin. To ensure you're getting the calcium, buy sardines that still contain the bones. Just like in salmon, these bones are edible and soft enough that you may not even notice them.

Sardines are also touted for their tryptophan, the essential amino acid important for synthesizing serotonin. Vitamin B_6 is found in high amounts in sardines, with one 3.75-ounce can providing about 18 percent of the current recommended daily value. This B vitamin is necessary for serotonin and melatonin production.

Need just one more reason to start snacking on sardines? This little fish is a source of omega-3 fatty acids, important for a healthy heart. Atlantic and Pacific varieties of sardines offer greater than 1,000 milligrams of omega-3 fatty acids per serving according to the USDA National Nutrient Database for Standard Reference.

How and When to Enjoy

Often touted as one of the healthiest foods around the world, sardines can be used in a variety of ways and are convenient to enjoy since they are readily available in canned form in most grocery stores. The 2015–2020 *Dietary Guidelines for Americans* recommends that we consume at least two servings of seafood a week for the nutritional benefits.

Sardines are enjoyed regularly by cultures around the world. In the Philippines, for example, sardines are simmered in a spicy tomato sauce to create the dish Ginisang Sardinas. This nutrient-rich fish can be used in place of anchovies in recipes like pasta puttanesca or on top of pizza. For a quick breakfast, chop sardines

Add sardines to a leafy green Mediterranean-inspired salad.

Serve on toast along with mashed avocado and tomato.

Include sardines in pasta with simple ingredients like garlic, capers, and fresh lemon zest.

and add to toast along with mashed avocado, tomato, and black pepper.

History

In the early twentieth century, sardines were abundant and became a staple in the diets of millions of soldiers fighting in both World Wars. The sardine population experienced a major decline in 1945, which was originally thought to be a result of overfishing, but may have also been related to the natural population fluctuations that occur due to oceanographic changes. As a result, sardine fishing was halted from the mid-1960s through 1986, and in the early 1990s populations of sardines recovered.

Nutrition Facts

In addition to the nutritional benefits already discussed, sardines are also a source of protein, iron, vitamin D, and vitamin B_{12}. They also have low levels of methyl mercury, which is often a concern for parents of young children as well as pregnant women who want to continue eating seafood but worry about mercury content in fish. A 2-ounce portion of sardines canned in water with sea salt provides:

Calories	90
Fat	4 g
Protein	13 g
Sodium	200 mg
Fiber	0 g
Carbohydrates	0 g
Sugar	0 g

Spinach

Sleep and Health Benefits

This green leafy vegetable is a source of calcium, magnesium, and potassium, each of which serves many important roles in the body and can impact sleep, as well as electrolyte balance, blood pressure, and bone health. According to the 2015–2020 *Dietary Guidelines for Americans*, potassium and calcium are two commonly under consumed nutrients for most people. Potassium and magnesium both help with muscle cramping, while calcium is important for melatonin production. Magnesium also plays a role in transporting calcium and potassium, demonstrating just how essential each of these nutrients are to one another.

Spinach is 91 percent water, so it will also contribute to your hydration needs throughout the day while providing a variety of nutrients. This leafy green is a source of iron, fiber, folate, vitamin K, and vitamin A.

How and When to Enjoy

We know Popeye loved the stuff, but spinach doesn't always receive rave reviews, especially from those who have only experienced eating poorly seasoned spinach straight from the can. Whether it's fresh, canned, or frozen, there are a number of ways that spinach can be used in recipes. Baby spinach has become a popular leafy green to make salads but can also be mixed in with other greens for color and texture variety. Enjoy fresh spinach sautéed lightly in butter with garlic or add some into omelets, soups, pasta dishes, or grain salads. You can even blend spinach into smoothies. Frozen spinach is good to keep on hand because it lasts longer than fresh and can easily be used in many of the same ways listed for fresh, except for making salads.

The texture of canned spinach is very different from fresh but can be used in lasagna and soups or mixed into meatloaf for a boost

Use baby spinach as a base for **salad** or mix with romaine for some variety in texture.	Add fresh spinach to smoothies for a serving of vegetables.
Include spinach in wraps or as a sandwich topping.	

of vegetables. Be sure to drain canned spinach well before using.

To extend the shelf life of fresh spinach, line either an airtight container or a resealable plastic bag with paper towels and add the greens. The greens should last seven to ten days in the refrigerator.

Calories	14
Fat	0 g
Protein	2 g
Sodium	47 mg
Fiber	1 g
Carbohydrates	2 g
Sugar	0 g

History

Spinach is believed to have originated in ancient Persia, making its way to China around A.D. 650. Catherine de' Médici, the queen of France in the sixteenth century, enjoyed spinach so much that she had her chefs prepare it at almost every meal. *Florentine* is used in the names of some dishes with spinach; the descriptor is a nod to her Florence birthplace.

Nutrition Facts

Spinach is low in calories and naturally fat-free and cholesterol-free. In a 2-cup serving of raw spinach you will get:

Strawberries

Sleep and Health Benefits

This much-loved berry provides the body with potassium, an essential nutrient for balancing electrolytes and aiding in muscle contractions. In addition, diets rich in potassium can help reduce blood pressure and the risk for stroke. Many American adults are falling short of the daily adequate intake level for potassium of 4,700 milligrams for women and men ages nineteen to fifty years old.

Strawberries are 91 percent water, which makes them a hydrating food choice that helps you get closer to your daily hydration needs. Research suggests that enjoying a serving of eight strawberries a day could help reduce the risk of heart disease and cancer and help manage diabetes. Strawberries are an excellent source of immune-boosting vitamin C, containing more vitamin C in a 1-cup serving than is found in one small orange! They also are a source of folate and are naturally fat-free and high in fiber.

How and When to Enjoy

Strawberries are at their peak in the early summer months. To choose the best berries, look for a bright red color with green leaves. Keep fresh strawberries in the refrigerator, and do not rinse them until ready to eat to prevent the berries from getting mushy. When ready to enjoy, rinse the strawberries and then pat dry with a paper towel before removing the leaves and stem with a paring knife.

Fresh strawberries make a great snack or addition to any meal! You can also top leafy green salads with sliced strawberries for a hint of sweetness, or add them to yogurt or cottage cheese for a protein-rich breakfast. Make a fresh fruit salsa by combining diced strawberries, kiwi, mango, and a squeeze of lime juice and serve over grilled fish or with pita chips for a refreshing summer snack. Frozen and freeze-dried strawberries are also nutritious options and can easily be added to smoothies, oatmeal, and cereal.

To satisfy a sweet tooth, have fresh strawberries topped with a dollop of whipped cream.

Start the day with a serving of strawberries paired with yogurt and pistachios.

Have strawberries with string cheese or a handful of almonds for a balanced snack.

History

The Romans used strawberries medicinally to alleviate melancholy, kidney stones, and a wide variety of illnesses. The strawberry has long been used as a symbol of love due to its color and heart shape. Today, California produces the majority of the strawberry crop in the United States, and Americans love this summer berry so much that one-third of US consumers chose strawberries as their favorite fruit in a 2016 survey conducted by the California Strawberry Commission.

On average, there are two hundred tiny seeds on every strawberry.

Nutrition Facts

One cup of whole strawberries, or approximately eight medium strawberries, will provide:

Calories	46
Fat	0 g
Protein	1 g
Sodium	1 mg
Fiber	3 g
Carbohydrates	11 g
Sugar	7 g

Sunflower Seeds

Sleep and Health Benefits

Sunflower seeds contain vitamin B_6, the nutrient involved in over 100 enzyme reactions, including supporting nerve function and helping to convert tryptophan into serotonin and eventually melatonin. A deficiency of vitamin B_6 has been associated with feelings of sadness, depression, anxiety, and increased feelings of pain, all of which can disrupt healthy sleep cycles. In a ¼-cup serving of sunflower seeds you'll find approximately 0.27–0.48 milligrams of vitamin B_6. These little seeds are also a source of magnesium, which aids in decreasing inflammation and muscle cramping, and may help lower stress levels and contribute to healthy thyroid function. Normal levels of magnesium have also been linked to better mental health.

If you're trying to include more fiber in your diet, try adding a serving of sunflower seeds. It's easy to incorporate them into different dishes, and the increased fiber content will only help you to feel more satisfied after a meal or a snack. In addition to fiber, these tiny seeds pack plenty of nutritional benefits, including being a source of healthy fats, iron, zinc, folate, vitamin E, and phosphorus.

How and When to Enjoy

Sunflower seeds are available in the shell or hulled, raw, dry-roasted, oil-roasted, salted, flavored, or unsalted. Besides snacking on them straight from the bag, they can be used as a topping for salads, oatmeal, yogurt, cereal, and homemade baked goods. If you like making homemade granola bars or energy bites, these seeds can easily be included. Sunflower seed butter, similar to peanut butter, has also become easier to find in grocery stores and is a great alternative for those with a peanut allergy. Sunflower seeds can also be used to make pesto in place of the usual pine nuts suggested in pesto recipes.

Mix sunflower seeds into oatmeal, cereal, or yogurt.

Sunflower seeds make a great addition to homemade trail mix.

Use sunflower seeds as a topping for home-made baked goods to provide a nutritional boost.

It's best to keep raw sunflower seed kernels in an airtight container in a cool, dry place up to three months. Seeds still in the shell can be kept up to a year.

History

Sunflower seeds have a history going back to 3000 B.C. when Native Americans used them to make flour for bread, and they ate the seeds as we still do today. The sunflower is thought to be named so because of its resemblance to the sun and for how the head of the plant follows the sun throughout the day. Ukraine and Russia are the current top sunflower seed producers in the world. In the United States, California, Minnesota, and North Dakota are top producers.

Nutrition Facts

By weight, sunflower seeds are made up of 47 percent fat and 24 percent protein. A ¼-cup portion of sunflower seeds provides:

Calories	53
Fat	5 g
Protein	2 g
Sodium	15 mg
Fiber	1 g
Carbohydrates	2 g
Sugar	0 g

Sweet Potatoes

Sleep and Health Benefits

Potassium is the showcase nutrient in sweet potatoes when it comes to sleep since potassium can help ease muscle cramping and regulate water balance. If your diet is lacking in potassium like most American diets, then include a serving of this potassium-rich tuber into your weekly meal plan. One medium sweet potato, about 5" in length, contains 438 milligrams of potassium.

There are about 0.6 milligrams of vitamin B_6 in ½ cup of mashed sweet potatoes. Vitamin B_6 is essential for protein metabolism and helping convert tryptophan into serotonin and eventually melatonin. As a complex carbohydrate, sweet potatoes are a good source of fiber, so they'll keep you feeling fuller longer after a meal. High-fiber foods tend to take longer to eat, allowing the stomach the time it needs to release leptin (the "appetite suppressor") and signal to the brain that you are full, preventing overeating at a meal.

This orange tuber is also high in vitamin A and vitamin C, both of which play an important role in immune system health, and it is fat-free and cholesterol-free.

While sweet potatoes are often referred to as *yams* and vice versa, they are from different botanical families and are not the same.

How and When to Enjoy

Sweet potatoes can be roasted whole, cubed, or as wedges like fries. Mashed sweet potatoes are equally nutritious as whole sweet potatoes and work well as a side dish in place of regular potatoes. Canned and frozen varieties of sweet potatoes are also available.

Diced or cubed sweet potatoes work well as a side dish, added to frittatas, as a salad topping, or mixed into grain-based salads. Shredded sweet potatoes can be used similarly to white

Try a loaded baked sweet potato as an easy meal, like the Loaded Southwest Sweet Potatoes in Chapter 4.

Roast cubed sweet potatoes with olive oil and chili powder for a flavorful side dish.

Add diced sweet potatoes to leafy green salads.

potatoes to make potato pancakes; serve with a savory or sweet yogurt-based dip.

When buying sweet potatoes, look for those that are small to medium in size and have unbruised skins. Store them in a cool, dark, and dry area and use within a week of purchase.

History

The sweet potato originated in Central and South America and is a member of the morning glory plant family. Unlike the name may imply, sweet potatoes are not related to the potato, which is a member of the Solanaceae family. Consumption of this tuber has grown nearly 42 percent from 2000 to 2016, and North Carolina has been the top producer of sweet potatoes in the US since 1971, producing nearly 60 percent of the sweet potatoes that were grown in 2015.

Nutrition Facts

One medium sweet potato, about 5" in length, provides:

Calories	100
Fat	0 g
Protein	2 g
Sodium	5 mg
Fiber	4 g
Carbohydrates	33 g
Sugar	7 g

Tart Cherries

Sleep and Health Benefits

This summer stone fruit naturally contains melatonin, the hormone that regulates the body's internal clock. Tart cherries are one of the few foods that contain melatonin, and researchers believe that it's the combination of melatonin and procyanidins and anthocyanins—two types of polyphenols—in cherries that helps improve sleep. The Montmorency variety of cherries have a sweet-sour taste and have been studied in depth for their health benefits.

In a 2018 randomized, double-blind, placebo-controlled pilot study published in the *American Journal of Therapeutics*, Montmorency tart cherry juice was found to help prolong sleep by 84 minutes in a group of eight study participants ages fifty and older who reported suffering from insomnia. The individuals in the group who drank Montmorency cherry juice consumed 8 fluid ounces of juice twice each day, once in the morning and 1–2 hours before bedtime, for fourteen days.

The signature ruby red color and tartness of cherries is attributed to anthocyanins. This tiny fruit has been researched and credited for relieving arthritis and gout symptoms and reducing muscle soreness after workouts, in addition to its sleep-promoting qualities. A ½-cup serving of frozen tart cherries is also a good source of vitamin A and also provides a small amount of vitamin C, iron, and calcium.

How and When to Enjoy

June and July are peak months for fresh cherries in America. For the other ten months of the year when fresh cherries are not so readily available, tart cherry juice, dried cherries, or frozen cherries can be substituted.

Whether you prefer to enjoy them fresh or dried, cherries make for a nutritious snack. Dried fruits will always contain more natural sugar per ounce than their fresh counterparts since the water has

Choose dried Montmorency tart cherries as a snack an hour before bedtime.

Include an 8-fluid-ounce glass of tart cherry juice at breakfast.

Pair dried tart cherries with almonds or walnuts for a satisfying, balanced snack.

been removed, making the sugar more concentrated. It's important to be mindful of serving sizes with all foods, but it can be easy to overconsume dried fruits since the recommended portion is only ¼ cup. For a balanced and more satisfying snack, I recommend pairing dried cherries with ¼ cup of walnuts or almonds to help stabilize blood sugars and to provide protein and heart-healthy fats to keep you feeling fuller longer.

Cooking with cherries? Think beyond pies, cobblers, and crisps! Cherries work well as a topping for oatmeal, yogurt parfaits, and grain salads such as quinoa. They can also be used in a savory-sweet sauce paired with grilled meats.

It's recommended to enjoy this tiny stone fruit an hour before bedtime for the best results.

History
Cherries have been relished for centuries around the globe and arrived in America with early settlers in the 1600s. The first cherry orchards planted for commercial purposes were in Michigan in the late 1800s, and the northern part of the state still remains one of the top cherry-producing regions in the country, growing about 75 percent of the tart cherry crop. The sweeter varieties of cherries such as Bing, Rainier, and Lambert are mostly grown in Oregon and Washington.

Nutrition Facts
The nutrition facts will vary between fresh, frozen, dried, canned, and tart cherry juice. The following nutrition facts are based on an 8-fluid-ounce serving of 100 percent tart cherry juice (with no added sugar):

Calories	140
Fat	0 g
Protein	1 g
Sodium	15 mg
Fiber	<1 g
Carbohydrates	34 g
Sugar	25 g

Tofu

Sleep and Health Benefits

Tofu often gets the reputation of being flavorless, and many bad experiences involving tofu revolve around negative thoughts about the texture. I've had my experiences with unpalatable tofu, but I've also had delicious tofu dishes! If you feel like there's no hope for this soy-based product, consider giving it another try in a new way so you can benefit from the sleep benefits tofu has to offer.

Tofu naturally contains calcium from the soybeans, but some soy foods are also fortified with calcium, which could offer additional sleep benefits since calcium is important for melatonin production. Firm tofu prepared with calcium sulfate, for example, contains about 568 milligrams of calcium per ⅓-cup serving. That's close to 50 percent of the recommended daily value for calcium! Additionally, magnesium chloride is usually added during processing to give tofu a smoother texture so you'll also be getting a source of magnesium from a serving of tofu.

How and When to Enjoy

Tofu may be something you've tried in the past and decided to never try again based on a bad experience. I hope that I can encourage you to give it another shot because when prepared correctly and used in the right recipes, it can taste great.

Often used as a high-protein, vegetarian alternative to meat, this soy-based product can easily find its place in any type of diet. There are different types of packaged tofu available in most grocery stores, including silken, firm, soft, and extra-firm. For smoothies, soups, or other recipes where a creamy consistency is desired, soft or silken tofu works best. Otherwise, firm or extra-firm tofu may be preferred. When using firm or extra-firm tofu, it's typically recommended to remove as much water as possible before cooking to get a crispier texture. In Chapter

Incorporate silken tofu into smoothies for a boost of protein.

Try the Tofu Spring Rolls with Carrot Ginger Sauce in Chapter 4.

Use tofu in a stir-fry recipe as an alternative source of protein.

4, you'll find several recipes that include tofu along with preparation tips. Tofu should be kept in the refrigerator until ready to use. If you find yourself with unused tofu, store it in an airtight container covered in filtered water and use within three days, being sure to change the water daily to maintain the freshness of the tofu.

History

Commonly referred to as *soybean curd*, tofu is made from curdled soy milk that is extracted from ground cooked soybeans. While the history of tofu reaches back centuries in Asian countries, it took most of the twentieth century for it to garner much interest from Americans. The United States is one of the largest producers of soybeans in the world, but tofu still is not widely consumed in America compared to other countries.

Nutrition Facts

Tofu is naturally cholesterol-free and is low in saturated fat. There are many types of tofu, and because they're processed in different ways, the nutrition facts will vary. Check the Nutrition Facts label when purchasing tofu products. A ⅓-cup serving of firm tofu provides approximately:

Calories	120
Fat	7 g
Protein	14 g
Sodium	12 mg
Fiber	2 g
Carbohydrates	2 g
Sugar	0 g

Tomatoes

Sleep and Health Benefits

Botanically recognized as a fruit, the tomato offers several sleep-promoting qualities, including being a source of potassium and melatonin and having a high water content. The tomato is approximately 94 percent water, contributing to the body's daily hydration needs.

This summer favorite is one of the few melatonin-containing foods. Melatonin not only helps to regulate your sleep-wake cycles; it has also been shown to be involved in a number of biological and physiologic functions, including gastrointestinal and cardiovascular health through the antioxidant effects of melatonin.

The potassium in tomatoes helps alleviate muscle cramping and is essential for water balance in the body. Potassium is one of the top nutrients lacking in the American diet, and 1 cup of cherry tomatoes contains 353 milligrams of potassium, which is nearly 8 percent of the daily adequate intake goal for men and women ages nineteen and up.

In addition, the antioxidant lycopene is found in tomatoes along with vitamin C, which is important for skin health and immune health.

How and When to Enjoy

Red, yellow, green, or purple, there are endless choices when choosing tomatoes and just as many ways to use them. Tomatoes can be enjoyed raw, roasted, stewed, sun-dried, simmered into a sauce, or added into a variety of recipes.

The process of cooking tomatoes actually enhances the absorption of lycopene, so go ahead and stock the pantry with canned tomato products and drink that glass of tomato juice for breakfast! Canned tomato products are convenient to keep on hand when you want to make a soup, chili, pasta, or a number of other recipes.

If you experience gastroesophageal reflux, tomato products may not be suitable if your

Include grape tomatoes or cherry tomatoes in leafy green salads or grain-based salads.

Enjoy whole-grain pasta with a marinara sauce.

Add sliced tomatoes to sandwiches and wraps.

reflux symptoms are triggered by acidic foods and beverages. Reflux symptoms are typically triggered by tomato sauces or foods that use it, such as pizza and chili, so fresh tomatoes may not be an issue, but it's best to determine what foods cause you to experience symptoms.

History

While many people probably associate tomatoes with Mediterranean cuisine, they actually evolved on a completely different hemisphere. The first tomatoes originated in the area we know now as Peru. When tomatoes made their way over to Spain, many people thought they were poisonous, capable of turning the blood into acid if you ate one, due to the resemblance of the tomato plants to deadly nightshade. In the 1900s, tomatoes finally started to gain acceptance in America, especially after the Campbell Soup Company invented the condensed tomato soup in 1897.

Nutrition Facts

Tomatoes are a low-calorie, low-carbohydrate, and fat-free food. A 1-cup serving of raw cherry tomatoes provides the following:

Calories	27
Fat	0 g
Protein	1 g
Sodium	7 mg
Fiber	2 g
Carbohydrates	6 g
Sugar	4 g

Top Sirloin Steak

Sleep and Health Benefits

Top sirloin steak is versatile and easy to prepare, and it offers several nutritional benefits. Beef is an excellent source of vitamin B_6, the vitamin important for serotonin and melatonin production, along with numerous other functions in the body. With 0.5 milligrams of vitamin B_6 in a 3-ounce serving of cooked top sirloin steak, this one serving will provide close to 38 percent of the vitamin's current recommended daily allowance.

Research has shown that having 25–30 grams of protein at meals can help with weight maintenance or weight loss, can improve satiety, and may prevent overconsumption of snacks in between meals. In a small, randomized study published in 2016 in the *American Journal of Clinical Nutrition*, researchers found that the consumption of a higher-protein diet, approximately 30 percent of total calories, may improve sleep in overweight and obese adults.

Additionally, top sirloin steak also provides zinc, iron, vitamin B_{12}, and choline.

How and When to Enjoy

Often one of the less expensive cuts of beef, top sirloin steak is great for grilling, stir-frying, broiling, or skillet cooking. Try adding cooked top sirloin steak to leafy green salads, pasta, and sandwiches, or serve it over quinoa with roasted vegetables for a Mediterranean-inspired meal. You can even add sliced top sirloin steak to an English muffin with a cooked egg and fresh spinach for a satisfying breakfast option.

When choosing top sirloin steaks, opt for those that have had most of the visible fat already removed to save you time trimming it at home before preparing. Beef should be kept refrigerated until ready to cook—there's no need to bring it to room temperature beforehand, no matter what cooking method you decide to use.

Add top sirloin steak to stir-fries and serve over brown rice.

Use seasoned top sirloin steak in tacos.

Use leftover top sirloin steak on breakfast sandwiches for a protein-packed start to the day.

To save money at the meat case, buy top sirloin steaks in family-sized packs. If you plan to save some of the steaks to use later, divide them and wrap the ones to be frozen in parchment paper before placing them into a resealable freezer bag. Use within one year, and unthaw completely in the refrigerator before cooking. Top sirloin steak does not have to be marinated in order to tenderize it, which makes it a great option for quick meals during the busy week.

It's best to enjoy higher-protein meals at least 3–4 hours before going to bed to allow for optimal digestion.

History

While cattle have been present in America since the mid-1500s, it wasn't until the Civil War when supplies of chicken and pork became depleted that people began demanding beef. Over the past thirty years, America's beef supply has become leaner due to breeding of leaner cattle, changes

in feeding practices, and trimming of fat before the product reaches consumers in grocery stores. The top sirloin steak is cut from the dorsal part of the sirloin primal cut section of beef cattle. Today, the states with the most cattle include Texas, Nebraska, and Kansas.

Nutrition Facts

Fresh beef is naturally low in sodium and high in protein. The fat content will vary depending on the cut of beef, but top sirloin steak is a lean cut of beef according to the USDA guidelines for lean meat. A 3-ounce portion of cooked top sirloin steak, trimmed of visible fat, contains:

Calories	180
Fat	8 g
Protein	25 g
Sodium	52 mg
Fiber	0 g
Carbohydrates	0 g
Sugar	0 g

Tuna

Sleep and Health Benefits

Similar to salmon and sardines, tuna is a source of vitamin B_6. Yellowfin tuna has the highest concentration of vitamin B_6 of all seafood sources, providing about 1 gram in a 4-ounce raw portion. Getting adequate amounts of this B vitamin is essential for a variety of functions in the body, but specifically the production of serotonin and melatonin helps the body rest peacefully at night. Tuna also contains tryptophan, the amino acid that is required for the creation of serotonin.

With about 40 milligrams of magnesium per 4-ounce serving, yellowfin tuna is a good source of this mineral that can decrease stress levels, inflammation, muscle cramping, and the occurrence of migraines.

Another great health benefit of eating tuna is the omega-3 fatty acid content. Studies have shown that diets rich in omega-3 fats can help reduce the risk of depression, heart disease, dementia, and arthritis.

How and When to Enjoy

There are a number of tuna species, different methods of catching them, and a variety of sourcing locations around the world, so to make sustainable seafood choices check out the Monterey Bay Aquarium Seafood Watch program's "Best Choices" list at www.seafoodwatch.org or download their app. Current recommended tuna species include albacore, skipjack, and yellowfin (commonly referred to as *ahi*).

Canned seafood is typically the most budget-friendly option and is easy to keep in the pantry as a high-quality source of protein. Frozen seafood is also usually a good value, can be prepared quickly, and is just as nutritious as fresh seafood. It's best to thaw frozen fish in the refrigerator overnight.

For a lighter tuna salad, swap out mayonnaise for mashed avocado to add creaminess, or use a combination of avocado, plain Greek yogurt, and maybe a touch of sriracha for a little spiciness. This

Enjoy tuna for lunch with Zesty Tuna Lettuce Wraps in Chapter 4.

Get adventurous and try the popular Hawaiian dish tuna poke, made with raw tuna.

Keep canned tuna in the pantry to make easy weeknight meals.

makes for a great sandwich or wrap, a protein-rich salad topper, or a stuffing for low-carb lettuce wraps made with Bibb lettuce leaves.

Certain types of tuna may contain higher levels of mercury than others. The best choices for tuna, meaning they are safe to eat two to three servings a week, are varieties of canned light tuna such as skipjack tuna, while yellowfin tuna should be limited to one serving per week for pregnant women and children.

Remember, it's best to enjoy meals with a significant amount of protein at least 3–4 hours before going to bed to allow for optimal digestion. To aid in digestion, avoid lying down right after a meal.

History

The classic tuna sandwich that many Americans today grew up eating first made its appearance in the late nineteenth century, but it wasn't until canned tuna became available that home cooks started making tuna salad sandwiches.

Before we started turning tuna into sandwiches, tuna was viewed as a "scrap" fish, often used to make pet foods, but otherwise when caught it was tossed back into the ocean.

Nutrition Facts

Nutrition facts will vary depending on the type of tuna and whether it is raw, cooked, or canned. For canned tuna, the sodium content will be higher to start compared to raw or cooked tuna and is available canned in either water or olive oil, which will impact total fat content. A 4-ounce portion of raw yellowfin tuna provides:

Calories	124
Fat	1 g
Protein	28 g
Sodium	51 mg
Fiber	0 g
Carbohydrates	0 g
Sugar	0 g

Turkey

Sleep and Health Benefits

Of all the foods that can help you sleep, turkey is probably the one that comes to mind first for most people. We've all heard that turkey is the cause of the "post-Thanksgiving-dinner-hangover nap," but how did it become the food we attribute that holiday snooze with?

The tryptophan in turkey usually gets blamed for sleepy feelings on Thanksgiving Day, but there are plenty of other foods that contain tryptophan. So what's the true cause of the extreme sleepy feeling after the Thanksgiving meal?

You can thank all the carbohydrates on the table—the mashed potatoes, marshmallow-covered yams, dinner rolls, and pies. When you eat carbs, insulin is released to help remove glucose from the bloodstream, but it also removes most of the amino acids from the blood, except for tryptophan. This is where turkey comes into play. Since tryptophan is left alone in the bloodstream without other amino acids to compete with, it can more freely cross the blood-brain barrier to help form serotonin and then, ultimately, melatonin.

To avoid the sluggish feeling after a meal, be sure to consume complex carbohydrates since they are digested slower than simple carbohydrates, and will prevent a large dose of insulin from being released in the bloodstream.

In addition to tryptophan, turkey has the important serotonin- and melatonin-producing nutrient, vitamin B_6. In a 3-ounce portion of roasted turkey, there's about 0.4 milligrams of the vitamin. Remember that vitamin B_6 is responsible for converting tryptophan into serotonin, which eventually leads to melatonin being produced.

How and When to Enjoy

Turkey can be enjoyed beyond Thanksgiving or as a deli meat sandwich. There are a number of different turkey cuts available, and more grocery stores are starting to carry a variety of them in the meat

Use cooked turkey breast tenderloins in homemade quesadillas.

Try turkey meatballs served over spaghetti with marinara sauce.

Serve pulled turkey in soups or on top of leafy green salads.

case. Some of the more commonly found turkey options are whole, ground, breast tenderloins, thighs, wings, meatballs, canned, and deli meat.

Ground turkey is made with both white and dark meat, and there are a number of options available at the supermarket with varying amounts of total fat ranging from 85–99 percent fat-free. If purchasing ground turkey, look for blends that contain 10 percent fat or less.

Food safety is always important to keep in mind, but it's especially important to be aware of salmonella when cooking poultry. Remember to keep turkey and any utensils used to prepare turkey separate from other foods and to wash hands and utensils thoroughly after touching the product. Turkey should always be cooked to an internal temperature of 165°F, tested with a meat thermometer. Keep turkey products refrigerated or frozen and be sure to refrigerate leftovers promptly.

History

Turkeys populated areas of the United States, Mexico, and Central America long before European settlers arrived. Many of today's domesticated turkeys are the Broad Breasted White variety, bred to produce a larger proportion of white meat since that's what most Americans prefer from the turkey. The top turkey-producing states in the US include Minnesota, North Carolina, Arkansas, and Indiana.

Nutrition Facts

Nutrition data will vary for different turkey products, so check the Nutrition Facts label to see specific information. A 4-ounce portion of turkey breast tenderloins provides:

Calories	100
Fat	2 g
Protein	21 g
Sodium	360 mg
Fiber	0 g
Carbohydrates	0 g
Sugar	0 g

Valerian Root Tea

Sleep and Health Benefits

As an herbal tea, valerian root is reported to help fight insomnia and may decrease anxiety and psychological stressors, although more research is needed in this area. Valerian root works similarly to a sedative, calming the central nervous system. Studies have shown that valerian root not only assists with falling asleep faster but also improves sleep quality. A randomized, triple-blind, controlled trial published in *Menopause* in 2011, found that an intervention group of fifty postmenopausal women experiencing insomnia benefited from taking valerian extract twice a day during a four-week period. A significant improvement in quality of sleep was reported by women in the intervention group.

While the research results on valerian can differ, overall many studies have shown that this herb can improve sleep quality when taken within 2 hours of going to bed. It may take anywhere from a week to four weeks before effects become noticeable. There is also some research showing a synergistic effect between valerian and other herbs, such as lemon balm. Many popular tea brands offer "sleepy time" teas that include valerian with other calming herbs.

How and When to Enjoy

Valerian root is available as a dietary supplement but can also be found in many herbal teas intended for promoting sleep. You can find valerian root tea or herbal teas that include valerian root in most grocery stores or health foods stores. If the tea contains any other ingredients, make sure that it is still caffeine-free. Other common ingredients included in tea blends along with valerian root include chamomile, peppermint, and lavender. Valerian root by itself can be a bit stinky and off-putting, so it's often combined with more pleasant-smelling herbs to improve palatability. Steep tea bags according to the package

Have a cup of valerian root tea 1–2 hours before bedtime.

Not a fan of tea? Valerian root is available as an herbal supplement but consult your physician before using.

Pair a cup of valerian root tea with one of the bedtime snacks in Chapter 4.

directions and enjoy 1–2 hours before bedtime. When making your own herbal tea bags or adding the dried herb to an infuser, it's commonly recommended to steep 2–3 grams in 8 fluid ounces of hot water for 10–15 minutes.

As with some herbal teas, it's best to consult your doctor before consuming since there may be medication interactions or side effects. If you are pregnant or breastfeeding, ask your doctor before consuming any herbal teas, as there currently is not enough information about their safety in this population.

Taking valerian root along with sedative medications or alcohol is not recommended because excessive drowsiness can be an issue.

History

Valerian root has been used for centuries in the Mediterranean region to help ease insomnia, nervousness, stress, and headaches. Native to Europe and Asia, the flower has been naturalized in North America. This perennial plant produces white, purple, or pink flowers, but the dried roots are what's used to make teas and tinctures.

Nutrition Facts

Unsweetened valerian root tea is calorie-free and does not contain any carbohydrates, fat, or cholesterol. One cup of valerian root herbal tea blend contains:

Calories	0
Fat	0 g
Protein	0 g
Sodium	0 mg
Fiber	0 g
Carbohydrates	0 g
Sugar	0 g

Walnuts

Sleep and Health Benefits

For a natural way of possibly boosting serotonin and melatonin levels, try adding walnuts into your diet. Walnuts contain tryptophan, the amino acid responsible for serotonin creation and ultimately melatonin production.

Walnuts are also a food source for the sleep-regulator melatonin. Although there has been limited research specifically about walnuts and how their melatonin content improves sleep, a study with rats published in *Nutrition* in 2005 found that blood concentrations of melatonin increased in the group that was fed walnuts.

Besides offering tryptophan and melatonin, this tree nut is a good source of magnesium, the mineral that helps decrease stress and inflammation. Walnuts provide about 44 milligrams of magnesium per 1-ounce serving.

If you need another reason to start eating more walnuts, here's one to consider! Walnuts are the only nut that is an excellent source of the plant-based omega-3 fat alpha-linolenic acid (ALA). A 1-ounce serving packs 2.5 grams of this heart-healthy polyunsaturated fat. Omega-3 fatty acids cannot be made in the body, so they must come from foods such as walnuts, salmon, flaxseed, and avocado.

Walnuts also offer fiber and phosphorus in addition to the other health benefits mentioned.

How and When to Enjoy

This tree nut can be included at any meal and is a great option for an easy travel snack. Enjoy walnuts whole or chopped in oatmeal, in trail mix, on top of cottage cheese or yogurt along with fruit, in salads, or in homemade breads. Walnuts can also be finely ground in a food processor to create a crunchy topping for seafood, like salmon or cod, or used to thicken sauces. Chopped walnuts work well when making homemade snack bars and energy bites as well.

English walnuts and black walnuts are the two most popular

Add walnuts to a homemade trail mix for fiber and healthy fats.	Top oatmeal or yogurt parfaits with chopped walnuts.	Use finely chopped walnuts as a coating for fish or other lean meats.

varieties of walnuts today. If buying walnuts still in their shell, look for those that are free of holes or cracks. These can be stored in a cool, dry place up to three months. Shelled walnuts, on the other hand, should be kept in the refrigerator or even the freezer, depending on when you plan to use them. Unopened and opened bags of walnuts can be stored up to six months in the fridge or up to a year in the freezer. Keeping walnuts cool during storage prevents the fat inside them from going rancid, creating an off-taste. To save money on nuts and to prevent food waste, buy them in the quantities you need from the bulk bin rather than in bags from the baking aisle.

History

Walnut trees date back to 7000 B.C. in ancient Persia, which is where they got their original nickname, "Persian walnut." It wasn't until walnuts began being traded in European countries that they became known as "English walnuts," despite never being grown commercially in England. In the 1860s, the first California-based commercial walnut operation began in Santa Barbara County. Today, California walnuts make up three-quarters of the supply traded worldwide.

Nutrition Facts

A 1-ounce portion of walnuts, about seven whole walnuts, is considered a serving and contains:

Calories	183
Fat	18 g
Protein	4 g
Sodium	1 mg
Fiber	2 g
Carbohydrates	4 g
Sugar	1 g

Watermelon

Sleep and Health Benefits

As the name suggests, watermelon is full of water—about 92 percent water, in fact. Adequate hydration throughout the day is an important factor for getting a night of great sleep. This tasty summer fruit has much more to offer nutritionally than just water, though. Watermelon also contains vitamin B_6 and potassium, two more nutrients that play a role in peaceful sleep. Vitamin B_6 helps maintain nerve function and breaks down proteins such as tryptophan, thereby aiding in the production of serotonin.

Potassium is essential for water balance and can minimize the occurrence of muscle cramps. If you've experienced muscle cramping that has jolted you awake in the middle of the night, you may need additional potassium in your diet. A 2-cup serving of diced watermelon provides about 340 milligrams of potassium.

Besides being a hydrating snack, watermelon is also high in vitamin C, and contains vitamin A and the antioxidant lycopene.

The first cookbook published in 1776 in the United States included a recipe for watermelon rind pickles.

How and When to Enjoy

Watermelon is in season during summer months, but sliced, packaged watermelon is usually available year-round in the grocery stores in the United States.

To pick a ripe watermelon, look for one that is symmetrical in shape, feels firm, and has a pale-yellow spot on the bottom. Watermelon, like most melons, should be heavy for its size, so lift it up to check this. It's best to wash watermelon before slicing into it to remove any germs that may be on the surface.

Keep a whole watermelon on the counter unless it was refrigerated when purchased, then store it in the refrigerator. Watermelon that has been cut should be kept in an airtight container or a sealed

Keep sliced water-melon on hand as an easy snack option.

Eat this hydrating summer fruit after a workout to replenish electrolytes.

Make homemade pop-sicles with fresh water-melon juice.

plastic bag in the fridge. It can easily absorb odors, so do not let cut watermelon sit open in the refrigerator.

This hydrating summer fruit works well in fruit salads, leafy green salads, and even grain salads. For a very hydrating beverage, infuse water with watermelon cubes in a pitcher and keep in the refrigerator. Before you throw away that rind, consider using it! It can be chopped and used in a stir-fry or sliced and pickled as is common in many southern states in the US.

History

Watermelon is in the same family as cucumbers, pumpkin, and squash. The first recorded harvest took place in Egypt nearly 5,000 years ago. Over 113,000 acres of watermelons were grown in 2017 across the United States, and the US currently ranks sixth in worldwide production. The top watermelon-producing states are Texas, Florida, Georgia, and California. The average watermelon consumption per capita is about 16 pounds per person, according to the Agricultural Marketing Resource Center.

Nutrition Facts

A 2-cup serving of diced water-melon provides approximately:

Calories	91
Fat	0 g
Protein	2 g
Sodium	3 mg
Fiber	1 g
Carbohydrates	23 g
Sugar	19 g

Whole-Grain Bread

Sleep and Health Benefits

Like brown rice and barley, whole-grain bread is a source of complex carbohydrates. It has more fiber than white bread per slice, so it keeps you feeling fuller longer and hopefully will prevent any middle-of-the-night snacking. Whole-grain bread contains more of the naturally occurring nutrients compared to refined white bread that has been processed, stripped of the germ, endosperm, and bran, then fortified to replace the nutrients that have been lost.

This carbohydrate food source also provides the body with vitamin B_6, the important nutrient for sleep. If you recall, vitamin B_6 is necessary for melatonin (the sleep-promoting hormone) and serotonin (the "happy neurotransmitter") production.

How and When to Enjoy

Since the endosperm, germ, and bran are left on the wheat, the bread often tastes nutty and has a denser texture than white bread.

To ensure you are getting all the benefits of whole-grain bread, read the ingredient list on the package and check that whole-wheat flour, or another whole grain, is listed as the first ingredient. If you live in Canada, *whole grain whole wheat* will be the term used.

Whole-grain breads can be enjoyed the same way white bread is used—make a grilled cheese, toast a slice for breakfast, or make French toast on the weekend.

Today, Kansas is the largest producer of wheat, producing enough in one year to bake 36 billion loaves of bread!

History

Bread as we know it today came about over centuries and thanks to several innovations, including bread leavening, refining flours, and mechanical slicing. The leavening of bread allowed us to move from flatbread like matzo, to fluffy, raised loaves. Yeast is the most common leavening agent;

Swap out white bread for whole-grain bread.

Use whole-grain bread crumbs in recipes when possible.

Try a slice of whole-grain toast topped with avocado and an egg for a filling breakfast.

yeast production for commercial purposes dates back to 300 B.C. in Egypt.

While very early bread makers would grind grains by hand and rock, the process of milling made it easier to create soft, finely ground flour. It was in 1917 that the first mechanized bread slicer was invented, but it took a while for this process to become standard practice. A little more than a decade after its invention, 90 percent of store-bought bread was presliced. Eventually, sliced white bread became the preferred choice, but as more and more consumers have learned about the nutritional benefits of whole-grain bread in recent years, and grown to appreciate its nutty taste, whole-grain breads have regained popularity.

Nutrition Facts

The nutrition information will vary slightly depending on the brand of whole-grain bread purchased, but the nutrition facts for one slice

of commercially made 100 percent whole-wheat bread are:

Calories	100
Fat	2 g
Protein	4 g
Sodium	130 mg
Fiber	2 g
Carbohydrates	19 g
Sugar	2 g

Whole-Grain Pasta

Sleep and Health Benefits

Similar to whole-wheat bread, whole-grain pastas are a source of complex carbohydrates. Compared to pasta made with white flour, whole-grain pasta will have a higher fiber content, making it a more filling and satisfying option that can help control ghrelin (the appetite-promoting hormone). Whole-grain foods have also been linked with improved blood sugar control after meals, which could help prevent sleep disturbances at night related to blood sugar spikes or dips. Pastas made with whole grains will also contain more of the naturally occurring nutrients, such as vitamin B_6, since the germ, endosperm, and bran are still present, rather than stripped away as they are when grains are refined. Remember, vitamin B_6 is necessary for nerve function and breaks down proteins such as tryptophan, thereby aiding in the production of serotonin (the "happy neurotransmitter") and melatonin (the sleep-promoting hormone).

How and When to Enjoy

When creating a meal with pasta, make the most of it by adding a variety of colorful ingredients! Pasta is a great vehicle for adding more vegetables to the plate—spinach, bell peppers, mushrooms, onions, tomatoes, carrots, and the list could go on and on. By including plenty of vegetables, you add lots of color to the plate, increase the "bulk" of the meal so you feel more satisfied, and get more nutritional value compared to just a plate of pasta covered with tomato sauce. You can also add a protein to the pasta dish or serve one alongside.

To limit the amount of saturated fat and cholesterol in pasta dishes, avoid butter sauces and cream-based sauces such as Alfredo, and be mindful of the amount of cheese being added.

As with whole-wheat bread, check the ingredient list to make

Use whole-grain spaghetti in place of refined-wheat spaghetti.

Ask for whole-grain pasta when dining out at restaurants.

Look for prepackaged whole-grain products like macaroni and cheese to replace the refined grain alternatives.

sure the pasta is made with 100 percent whole-wheat flour or whole-grain flour. The texture of whole-wheat pasta is often described as having more "tooth," or being slightly chewier. Whole-grain pasta can be used in place of white pasta, but it may require a slightly longer cooking time. Follow package directions to prepare whole-grain pasta appropriately. There are whole-grain varieties of most pasta shapes, including penne, elbow macaroni, and even lasagna noodles. Keep pasta stored in a dry place.

History

Pasta is an integral part of many different cuisines around the world and comes in many different forms. Durum wheat flour is what makes up traditional wheat-based pastas, and it's thought that this particular type of pasta originated in the Mediterranean region. The durum flour gave pasta a higher gluten content and a longer shelf life once dried. When Italian immigrants came to America in the late nineteenth century, pasta soon became a staple food in the United States.

Nutrition Facts

Pasta is another food where it's very easy to go overboard on appropriate portion sizes. The recommended serving size for most cooked pasta is anywhere from a ½–1 cup. Most restaurant pasta portions are at least double that amount and usually are not made with whole-grain pastas, although that option is being offered in more places now. A ⅔-cup serving of cooked, plain, whole-grain penne pasta will provide about:

Calories	200
Fat	2 g
Protein	7 g
Sodium	5 mg
Fiber	6 g
Carbohydrates	41 g
Sugar	2 g

Yogurt

Sleep and Health Benefits

Yogurt, whether it's regular yogurt or Greek, is a source of potassium, calcium, and magnesium. These three nutrients serve many purposes in the body, including impacting sleep, as well as electrolyte balance, blood pressure, and bone health. Calcium and potassium are two commonly under consumed nutrients for Americans, as noted in the 2015–2020 *Dietary Guidelines for Americans*. Potassium and magnesium can help with muscle cramping, while calcium is important for melatonin production. Magnesium also plays a role in transporting calcium and potassium, so you can see how all of these nutrients are integral to one another.

Certain yogurts include probiotics, healthy bacteria strains that we need for optimal gut health. The most common probiotic you'll find is lactobacillus, which is in yogurt and other fermented foods.

How and When to Enjoy

Remember the tips in the Nutrition Facts section on the following page when you head to the store to buy yogurt. The same applies to drinkable yogurts since many of these products can have excessive amounts of sugar. Making yogurt at home is also an option, and there are several great recipes online to get you started.

A cup of yogurt or a parfait at breakfast may be the more common way to enjoy this dairy food, but it's great at any time of day! It can be a satisfying sweet treat before bed if topped with fresh fruit. Plain Greek yogurt is a higher-protein alternative to sour cream. Try using it to top your baked potato or nachos, or make a yogurt-based dip with it. Yogurt can also be used in baking to reduce calories and fat from oils. It's best to follow a recipe that has been developed with yogurt as an ingredient or to experiment with replacing only a portion of the oil rather than completely omitting it.

Make a yogurt parfait layered with fresh or frozen fruit for breakfast.

Mix yogurt into oatmeal for extra creaminess and a protein boost.

Pack a yogurt cup as a snack option at work and pair it with a handful of almonds or walnuts.

History

Yogurt is one of the oldest fermented foods, dating back to 6000 B.C. Turkish immigrants brought yogurt to America in the 1700s, but it took more than 200 years for it to start hitting grocery store shelves. In 1947, Dannon introduced the first yogurt with fruit on the bottom, and the popularity has been on a steady incline since then.

Nutrition Facts

The nutrition facts will vary drastically among brands and depending on many variables, including if it's plain, flavored, Greek, fat-free, sugar-free, or made with cow's milk, soy milk, or coconut milk. Even as a dietitian who reads nutrition labels regularly, I find the yogurt section overwhelming. It's incredible to think about how the yogurt section at the grocery store has exploded over the past few years, and some of the options are considerably better than others.

My word of advice to you when standing in front of the mile-long yogurt section is to look for one that contains probiotics, sometimes listed as live active cultures, has less than 10 grams of sugar, and contains at least 12 grams of protein per 5.3-ounce container. I usually suggest choosing a low-fat or full-fat yogurt so that it's satisfying enough to last, especially if this is the only thing you're eating for breakfast. If you pair it with another food that provides fat, like a handful of nuts or a cooked egg, then choose a yogurt that meets your taste preferences.

Zucchini

Sleep and Health Benefits

Made up of 95 percent water, zucchini is another great food to include in your weekly diet to contribute to your hydration levels. As discussed in Chapter 2, adequate hydration is important for a night of restful sleep. This green summer squash is also rich in potassium, the nutrient that is essential for water balance and that can minimize the occurrence of muscle cramps. One cup of chopped zucchini has 324 milligrams of potassium, providing approximately 7 percent of the recommended daily intake for men and women ages nineteen to fifty years old.

In addition to these sleep-promoting benefits, zucchini provides the body with vitamin A and vitamin C, important for immune health and many other functions in the body, and with folate. Although folate deficiency is rare in the United States, low levels have been linked to depression, and those taking an antidepressant may not respond as well to the medication as those with normal folate levels. Folate needs are increased for women who are pregnant or could become pregnant, and for those who are breastfeeding.

How and When to Enjoy

Although zucchini is a summer vegetable, it's readily available year-round in supermarkets. This squash is versatile and can stand on its own as a sautéed veggie or can be used in soups, casseroles, pastas, stir-fries, and omelets; zucchini can also take the place of pasta as "zoodles." While it's usually eaten cooked, zucchini tastes great raw dipped in hummus or a veggie dip. Grilled zucchini is another delicious way to enjoy it! Try the recipe for Veggie-Stuffed Zucchini in Chapter 4. When selecting zucchini, choose one with green skin that has minimal blemishes. Keep zucchini stored in the refrigerator up to five days in the crisper drawer and wash before preparing it. Zucchini

Add zucchini to stir-fry dishes, pasta, or an omelet.

Try using frozen zucchini in smoothies for extra fiber, water, and nutrients.

Zucchini is a great vegetable to snack on raw and dip into hummus.

can be prepped ahead of time and stored sliced in an airtight container in the refrigerator until you're ready to cook it. Cooked zucchini can usually keep one to two days in an airtight container in the refrigerator.

History

Native to Mexico and South America, zucchini is a member of the same family as cucumbers and melons. The variety we know and consume today was developed in Italy in the nineteenth century. Peak season for zucchini is from May to August. California, Florida, Georgia, and Michigan are leaders in zucchini squash production in the United States. According to the Agricultural Marketing Resource Center, the United States imports the most squash in the world, much of which is imported from Mexico.

Nutrition Facts

Zucchini and other summer squash are harvested while in an immature state for best taste and while the rind is still edible. At less than 25 calories per serving, zucchini is a low-calorie, low-carb, fat-free food. A 1-cup serving of chopped zucchini provides:

Calories	21
Fat	0 g
Protein	2 g
Sodium	10 mg
Fiber	3 g
Carbohydrates	4 g
Sugar	3 g

Peaceful Sleep Summary

Now that you have made it through the list of fifty foods, it's clear to see that there are several key nutrient players involved in getting a good night's sleep. A diet that includes many of the foods in this list, while minimizing or monitoring intake of the foods listed in Chapter 2, can lead you back to the healthy, restful sleep you've been daydreaming about!

Overall, research is limited on how specific foods impact sleep, but there is research supporting the importance of specific nutrients and their role in promoting quality sleep. Food is always the best way to get the nutrients your body needs because it offers multiple nutrition benefits, whereas supplements are offering either a specific nutrient or several, like a multivitamin. Nutrient-dense foods offer an "entourage effect," meaning the whole food is greater than the sum of its parts. The synergistic work that occurs when you consume a variety of foods cannot be matched or replicated by individual vitamins and minerals. Remember, choose food first and then use supplements to fill in any nutritional gaps.

PART 3

A Quick-Start Plan to Better Sleep

Sleep Well Again: Recipes and Meal Plans

This is where we put all of the pieces we've covered so far and put them into action. Let's take what we know about nutrition and sleep and put it into practice with some delicious recipes. The total sugar amounts in these recipes includes both naturally occurring sugars and, where applicable, added sugars.

Chocolate Cherry Oatmeal 150
Greek Quinoa Breakfast Bowl 151
Egg on Avocado Toast
    with Salsa 152
Cucumber Tartine 153
Tropical Chickpea Walnut
    Quinoa Bowl 154
Almond Butter Jelly Smoothie 156
Banana and Walnut Trail Mix 157
Chocolate Banana Oat Bites 158
Blueberry Cottage
    Cheese Parfait 160
Zesty Tuna Lettuce Wraps 161
Greek Chicken Rice Bowl 162
Chickpea and Squash Slow
    Cooker Curry 163
Grapefruit Salmon Salad 164
Roasted Summer
    Vegetable Panzanella 166
Zucchini Ribbons with Chickpeas and
    Olive Oil 168
Berry Coconut Smoothie Bowl 169
Sheet Pan Salmon and Vegetables 170
Blackened Salmon Tacos 172
Sweet Potato Fiesta Salad 174
Loaded Southwest
    Sweet Potatoes 175
Tofu Patty Melt 176
Chocolate Cherry Smoothie 177
Tofu Spring Rolls with Carrot
    Ginger Sauce 178
Cauliflower Cranberry
    Superfood Salad 180
Veggie-Stuffed Zucchini 181

Dried tart cherries contain melatonin and have been studied in depth for their health benefits. The fiber from the oatmeal, dried cherries, and walnuts will help keep you feeling full and satisfied throughout the morning. Preparing this oatmeal with milk instead of water will make it creamier and will also add protein, calcium, vitamin D, and phosphorus.

Sleep-promoting ingredients	oats, milk, tart cherries, walnuts
Serves	1
Prep time	5 minutes
Cook time	5 minutes

Per Serving	
Calories	460
Fat	19 g
Protein	15 g
Sodium	65 mg
Fiber	2 g
Carbohydrates	60 g
Sugar	26 g

Chocolate Cherry Oatmeal

½ cup rolled oats
1 cup 1% milk
2 tablespoons dried tart cherries
2 tablespoons chopped walnuts
1 tablespoon mini dark chocolate chips

1 Prepare oats according to package directions using either milk or water.

2 Once cooked, add dried cherries, walnuts, and chocolate chips and stir. Serve immediately.

Greek Quinoa Breakfast Bowl

½ cup uncooked quinoa, rinsed
1 cup water
1 teaspoon salt-free garlic and herb seasoning
⅛ teaspoon salt
½ cup diced red bell pepper
2 tablespoons finely diced red onion
2 tablespoons feta cheese
2 large eggs
1 tablespoon fresh chopped basil (for garnish)
¼ teaspoon black pepper

1 Combine quinoa, water, garlic and herb seasoning, and salt in a small saucepan. Bring to a boil over high heat. Once boiling, reduce to a simmer, cover with a lid, and cook 15–20 minutes or until liquid is absorbed. Fluff with a fork and remove from heat. Allow to cool 10 minutes.

2 Add the red bell pepper, onion, and feta cheese and mix.

3 Either place in an airtight container and store in the refrigerator until ready to use or divide the quinoa into two separate bowls.

4 Prepare eggs as desired and add on top of the quinoa in the bowls. Before serving, garnish with basil and black pepper.

Quinoa isn't usually thought of as a breakfast item, but it makes for a very filling and fiber-rich start to the day. When you want a savory breakfast, try this Greek Quinoa Breakfast Bowl topped with a runny egg. The quinoa can be prepared ahead of time and reheated so there's minimal prep involved when you're short on time in the morning.

Sleep-promoting ingredients	quinoa, cheese, egg
Serves	2
Prep time	10 minutes
Cook time	30 minutes

Per Serving	
Calories	280
Fat	10 g
Protein	14 g
Sodium	300 mg
Fiber	5 g
Carbohydrates	34 g
Sugar	4 g

This is one of my go-to breakfast options in the morning because I always keep these staple ingredients on hand. Avocado toast is great, but adding a protein-rich egg on top is even better! For extra flavor, try it topped with a spoonful of red or green salsa and even a sprinkle of shredded sharp Cheddar cheese.

Sleep-promoting ingredients	whole-grain bread, egg, avocado, tomato
Serves	1
Prep time	2 minutes
Cook time	8 minutes

Per Serving	
Calories	240
Fat	14 g
Protein	11 g
Sodium	390 mg
Fiber	4 g
Carbohydrates	18 g
Sugar	4 g

Egg on Avocado Toast with Salsa

1 slice whole-grain bread
1 large egg
¼ medium ripe avocado, peeled, pitted, and sliced
2 tablespoons salsa

1 Place bread in toaster and toast to desired doneness. Meanwhile, heat a small skillet over medium heat. Add egg and cook until the white part is nearly set, then gently flip using a spatula. Continue to cook until egg has reached desired doneness (about 1 minute for over easy, 2 minutes for over medium, and 3 minutes for over hard).

2 Top toast with avocado slices and gently smash with the back of a fork. Add egg to the avocado toast and top with salsa.

Cucumber Tartine

1 slice sprouted whole-grain bread
2 tablespoons feta cheese
1 tablespoon part-skim ricotta cheese
½ small cucumber, cut into very thin slices
Pinch salt

1 Place bread in toaster or toaster oven and toast as desired. Meanwhile, in a small bowl, mash together the feta cheese and ricotta cheese.

2 Spread the cheese mixture over the toast. Top with cucumber slices. Sprinkle with a pinch of salt.

With hydrating cucumbers, whole-grain bread, and feta and ricotta cheeses, every ingredient in this recipe will provide your body with what it needs for a restful night. This is a no-cook recipe and can easily be assembled at work for an easy lunch. Enjoy this dish with a serving of strawberries or watermelon for a balanced, filling meal.

Sleep-promoting ingredients	whole-grain bread, cheese, cucumber
Serves	1
Prep time	10 minutes
Cook time	N/A

Per Serving	
Calories	170
Fat	6 g
Protein	9 g
Sodium	270 mg
Fiber	4 g
Carbohydrates	22 g
Sugar	3 g

This recipe is bursting with fresh flavors and nourishing ingredients! Walnuts are the perfect choice for this recipe because they give a nice crunch and they're roasted in the oven, which enhances the depth of flavor. I use a store-bought coconut mango dressing for a tropical flavor, but you could also use light ranch dressing.

Sleep-promoting ingredients	quinoa, chickpeas, walnuts, avocado
Serves	2
Prep time	15 minutes
Cook time	30 minutes

Per Serving	
Calories	660
Fat	38 g
Protein	20 g
Sodium	480 mg
Fiber	17 g
Carbohydrates	68 g
Sugar	20 g

Tropical Chickpea Walnut Quinoa Bowl

⅓ cup quinoa
1 cup water
2 tablespoons olive oil
2 teaspoons sriracha
4 cups broccoli florets
1 cup canned chickpeas, drained and rinsed
½ cup chopped walnuts
¼ cup fat-free Sprouts Organic Coconut Mango dressing
1 medium red bell pepper, seeded and sliced thin
½ small avocado, peeled, pitted, and sliced
¼ cup fresh chopped cilantro
2 fresh lime wedges

1 Preheat oven to 450°F. Spray a baking sheet with cooking spray.

2 In a small saucepan over high heat, combine the quinoa and water and bring to a boil. Once boiling, reduce to a simmer, cover with a lid, and cook 15–20 minutes or until liquid is absorbed. Fluff with a fork and remove from heat.

3 Whisk together the olive oil and sriracha in a small bowl.

4 Add the broccoli to a large bowl and pour the sriracha olive oil over top and stir well to coat. Spread the broccoli onto the baking sheet and roast in oven 10 minutes on the middle oven rack.

5 Stir broccoli around on baking sheet and add the chickpeas and walnuts. Place back in oven and roast 5 minutes. Remove from oven and set aside in a large bowl.

6 To assemble quinoa bowls: Divide the quinoa and the broccoli, chickpeas, and walnuts between two bowls. Top each bowl with 2 tablespoons Coconut Mango dressing, red bell pepper, avocado, cilantro, and a fresh lime wedge.

Almond butter was used in this recipe since it contains less saturated fat than peanut butter, but you can use whatever nut butter you have on hand. The chia seeds provide heart-healthy omega-3 fatty acids, and while there are 14 grams of total fat, they're mostly monounsaturated and polyunsaturated fats (a.k.a. the good kind!). This truly tastes like a classic PB&J in smoothie form! You can also top this with additional frozen cherries and wild blueberries if desired.

Sleep-promoting ingredients	yogurt, tart cherries, almond butter
Serves	1
Prep time	5 minutes
Cook time	N/A

Per Serving	
Calories	360
Fat	14 g
Protein	12 g
Sodium	120 mg
Fiber	11 g
Carbohydrates	47 g
Sugar	30 g

Almond Butter Jelly Smoothie

4 fluid ounces 100 percent tart cherry juice
2 ounces 2% milk-fat Greek vanilla yogurt
½ cup frozen pitted dark sweet cherries or tart cherries
¼ cup frozen wild blueberries
1 tablespoon almond butter
1 tablespoon chia seeds

1 Combine all ingredients in a blender and process until smooth.

2 Pour into a glass and enjoy.

Banana and Walnut Trail Mix

½ cup walnut halves
½ cup banana chips
¼ cup dark chocolate–covered blueberries
2 tablespoons raw pumpkin seed kernels
2 tablespoons salted sunflower seeds

1 Combine all of the ingredients in a small bowl and mix.

2 Store in an airtight container or a Mason jar for up to two weeks at room temperature.

With potassium-rich banana chips and heart-healthy walnuts, this simple trail mix recipe will give you the energy your body needs to get through the day with all of the added nutrition benefits! Making your own trail mix is more affordable than buying it premade, plus you can customize it with ingredients you enjoy.

Sleep-promoting ingredients	walnuts, banana chips, pumpkin seed kernels, sunflower seeds
Serves	4
Prep time	5 minutes
Cook time	N/A

Per Serving	
Calories	240
Fat	19 g
Protein	5 g
Sodium	75 mg
Fiber	2 g
Carbohydrates	14 g
Sugar	9 g

These Chocolate Banana Oat Bites taste just like banana bread but with a bit of dark chocolate goodness! This is a good way to get your chocolate fix in a healthy and satisfying way. With oats, banana, almonds, and dark chocolate, you'll be getting lots of nutritional benefits to help promote good sleep.

Sleep-promoting ingredients	oats, banana, almonds, almond butter
Serves	7
Prep time	80 minutes
Cook time	N/A

Per Serving

Calories	210
Fat	11 g
Protein	5 g
Sodium	5 mg
Fiber	3 g
Carbohydrates	23 g
Sugar	10 g

Chocolate Banana Oat Bites

1 cup quick-cooking oats
1 medium ripe banana
¼ cup whole raw almonds
2 tablespoons unsweetened coconut flakes
1 tablespoon shelled hemp seeds
1 tablespoon almond butter (or other nut butter)
½ teaspoon ground cinnamon
½ cup dark chocolate morsels

1 In a food processor, combine all of the ingredients except for the chocolate until they form into a ball.

2 Line a baking sheet with parchment paper or a silicon mat. Using a tablespoon measure or scoop, form 1" balls and place onto baking sheet.

3 To melt the chocolate, use a saucepan and a glass bowl that fits inside the saucepan without touching the bottom. Fill the saucepan ¼ full with water and place the glass bowl on top (the water should not touch the bottom of the bowl). Bring the water to a boil, then reduce to a simmer. Add chocolate morsels to the glass bowl and melt, stirring occasionally with a rubber scraper or metal spoon. Once chocolate is melted (it may take about 4–5 minutes), turn off the heat.

4 Using a toothpick, pick up one ball at a time and dip it halfway into the chocolate, then place back onto baking sheet. Continue this until each ball is dipped in chocolate.

5 Place baking sheet in the refrigerator 1 hour to allow the chocolate to harden.

6 Keep the bites refrigerated until ready to eat. Best enjoyed within two to three days.

Tired of yogurt parfaits? Try a cottage cheese parfait instead! You could swap the blueberries in the recipe for strawberries, bananas, cherries, or whatever fruit you prefer. Have breakfast waiting on you in the morning by preparing this recipe the night before. Layer all of the ingredients in a container and then in the morning, top it off with shredded wheat cereal, coconut flakes, and chia seeds.

Sleep-promoting ingredients	cottage cheese, whole-grain cereal
Serves	1
Prep time	5 minutes
Cook time	N/A

Per Serving	
Calories	330
Fat	11 g
Protein	24 g
Sodium	470 mg
Fiber	8 g
Carbohydrates	35 g
Sugar	16 g

Blueberry Cottage Cheese Parfait

2/3 cup low-fat cottage cheese

1 teaspoon ground cinnamon

½ cup frozen blueberries, thawed, divided

½ cup shredded wheat breakfast cereal, divided

2 tablespoons shredded coconut flakes, divided

2 teaspoons chia seeds, divided

1 In a small bowl, mix together cottage cheese and cinnamon.

2 In a Mason jar or glass, spoon ⅓ cup cottage cheese mixture into the container. Top with ¼ cup blueberries followed by ¼ cup shredded wheat cereal, 1 tablespoon shredded coconut, and 1 teaspoon chia seeds.

3 Repeat the layers with the remaining ingredients. Best enjoyed right away so cereal does not become soggy.

Zesty Tuna Lettuce Wraps

10 ounces tuna (canned in water), drained well
½ small ripe avocado, peeled, pitted, and
*   sliced*
1 tablespoon chopped cilantro leaves
¾ teaspoon sriracha plus 2 teaspoons for
*   topping*
¼ teaspoon Dijon mustard
⅛ teaspoon black pepper
6 leaves Bibb lettuce

Toppings
¼ cup shredded carrots
¼ cup diced cucumber

1 In a small bowl, combine the drained tuna, avocado, cilantro, ¾ teaspon sriracha, mustard, and black pepper. Mix well until there are no chunks of avocado.

2 Evenly divide tuna among each lettuce leaf and top with diced carrots, cucumber, and remaining sriracha. Serve immediately or store lettuce wraps in an airtight container up to 24 hours.

These Zesty Tuna Lettuce Wraps can be easily assembled in less than 15 minutes, and make a light and refreshing meal. To cut calories and boost heart-healthy monounsaturated fats, this recipe swaps the usual mayonnaise for avocado. Avocado helps bind the tuna salad together and gives it some creaminess without all of the saturated fat.

Sleep-promoting ingredients	tuna, avocado, cucumber
Serves	2
Prep time	15 minutes
Cook time	N/A

Per Serving	
Calories	260
Fat	9 g
Protein	38 g
Sodium	140 mg
Fiber	4 g
Carbohydrates	6 g
Sugar	1 g

This recipe is light but still filling, and I love all of the colorful veggie toppings! You can make your own cauliflower rice at home by chopping a head of cauliflower in a food processor until it resembles rice, or you can buy it in the freezer section at the grocery store. Feel free to customize the toppings and add extra vegetables or herbs for more color. Fresh dill would be a great addition to this dish!

Sleep-promoting ingredients	cauliflower, cucumber, cheese
Serves	2
Prep time	15 minutes
Cook time	10 minutes

Per Serving	
Calories	330
Fat	11 g
Protein	34 g
Sodium	650 mg
Fiber	3 g
Carbohydrates	23 g
Sugar	9 g

Greek Chicken Rice Bowl

2 (5-ounce) boneless, skinless chicken breasts
½ teaspoon dried oregano
½ teaspoon dried thyme
½ teaspoon garlic powder
¼ teaspoon black pepper
1 (12-ounce) bag frozen cauliflower rice

Toppings
½ cup diced red bell pepper
½ cup diced yellow bell pepper
½ cup sliced cucumbers
½ cup shredded carrots
¼ cup sliced green onions
¼ cup feta cheese
¼ cup Litehouse Foods Feta Dill Greek
 Yogurt dressing

1 Season both sides of each chicken breast with oregano, thyme, garlic powder, and black pepper.

2 Lightly coat a small grill pan or skillet with cooking spray and heat over medium heat. Add the chicken once pan is hot. Cook 8–10 minutes or until the internal temperature reaches 165°F.

3 While chicken is cooking, prepare the cauliflower rice per package directions. Once chicken has finished cooking, slice into strips.

4 Divide the cauliflower rice between two bowls and top with sliced cooked chicken, vegetables, feta cheese, and dressing.

Chickpea and Squash Slow Cooker Curry

1 (12-ounce) bag frozen diced butternut squash
2 teaspoons coconut oil
½ cup chopped yellow onion
1½ tablespoons curry powder
1 teaspoon crushed red pepper
½ teaspoon ground turmeric
½ teaspoon salt
1 clove garlic, peeled and minced
1 (15-ounce) can chickpeas, drained and rinsed
2 cups roughly chopped lacinato kale
1 (14-fluid-ounce) can light coconut milk
½ cup frozen peas
8 fluid ounces vegetable broth
2 cups cooked brown rice or quinoa
¼ cup chopped cilantro, for garnish

1 Thaw squash according to package directions.

2 Heat coconut oil in a large skillet over medium heat for 1 minute. Add onions and cook 3 minutes before adding squash, curry powder, crushed red pepper, turmeric, salt, and garlic. Mix with spatula and allow to cook 3 minutes.

3 Pour squash mixture into a slow cooker, then add remaining ingredients except rice and cilantro. Cook on low 4–5 hours. Serve over ½ cup brown rice. Garnish with chopped cilantro.

This is a mild yellow curry dish and includes several sleep-promoting foods, like chickpeas and brown rice or quinoa. Take a shortcut with this dish and use frozen brown rice! This is a really great recipe to add to the weekly meal prep list, and it reheats well for leftovers.

Sleep-promoting ingredients	chickpeas, quinoa/brown rice
Serves	4
Prep time	15 minutes
Cook time	4–5 hours

Per Serving	
Calories	450
Fat	14 g
Protein	13 g
Sodium	700 mg
Fiber	11 g
Carbohydrates	72 g
Sugar	11 g

This is a very satisfying salad full of fresh citrus flavor! The vitamin C in the homemade citrus dressing and grapefruit helps with iron absorption from the leafy greens and the salmon, helping your body make the most of the nutrients.

Sleep-promoting ingredients	orange juice, grapefruit juice, salmon, avocado, edamame, pumpkin seeds
Serves	2
Prep time	15 minutes
Cook time	10 minutes

Per Serving	
Calories	590
Fat	31 g
Protein	52 g
Sodium	220 mg
Fiber	9 g
Carbohydrates	27 g
Sugar	12 g

Grapefruit Salmon Salad

Citrus Vinaigrette (makes about ½ cup)
¼ cup fresh orange juice (about 1 small navel orange)
2 tablespoons fresh grapefruit juice
2 tablespoons extra-virgin olive oil
1 tablespoon minced cilantro
2 teaspoons white wine vinegar
1 teaspoon fresh lime juice
1 clove garlic, peeled and finely minced

Salad
2 (6-ounce) salmon fillets
⅛ teaspoon each salt and black pepper
1 teaspoon olive oil
5 ounces baby lettuce mix
1 medium grapefruit, cut into sections
½ medium avocado, peeled, pitted, and sliced thin
½ cup frozen shelled edamame, thawed
¼ cup thinly sliced red onion
2 tablespoons raw unsalted pumpkin seeds

1 Prepare the citrus vinaigrette by combining all ingredients in a small mixing bowl or liquid measuring cup. Whisk together and set aside.

2 Prep the salmon fillets by placing them skin side down on a plate. Pat with a paper towel to dry. Season with salt and pepper.

3 Heat a 10" skillet over medium-high heat. Once hot, add olive oil. Carefully place the salmon fillets skin side up in the skillet and reduce the heat to medium. Cook 4–5 minutes or until the salmon is cooked halfway through. Gently turn the salmon fillets over and continue to cook another 3–5 minutes. Once the fillets are cooked through, place them on a clean plate. The skin should now be easy to remove in one piece using a pair of tongs or fork.

4 Prepare the salads in two large salad bowls starting with the baby lettuce mix. Top with the grapefruit, avocado, edamame, red onion, and pumpkin seeds. Place one salmon fillet on top of each salad and add dressing as desired.

The most important part about making a panzanella (bread salad) is choosing a hearty bread. A whole-grain baguette is the perfect fit! You could use a stale loaf of bread in this recipe rather than buying fresh bread and drying it out in the oven, but either method works.

Sleep-promoting ingredients	whole-grain bread, tomato, zucchini, cheese
Serves	6
Prep time	15 minutes
Cook time	40 minutes

Per Serving	
Calories	270
Fat	19 g
Protein	10 g
Sodium	160 mg
Fiber	1 g
Carbohydrates	18 g
Sugar	6 g

Roasted Summer Vegetable Panzanella

1 whole-grain baguette, cut into 1" cubes
1/3 cup olive oil plus 2 tablespoons, divided
1 small red onion, peeled, quartered, and sliced
1 pint grape tomatoes, halved
2 medium zucchini, cut into half moons
1/4 teaspoon salt
1/4 teaspoon black pepper, divided
1/4 cup balsamic vinegar
1 teaspoon whole-grain mustard
4 cups arugula
1 cup cubed fresh mozzarella
1/2 cup packed basil leaves, chopped

1 Preheat oven to 275°F.

2 Arrange bread cubes on a baking sheet and drizzle with 1 tablespoon olive oil. Bake bread cubes 20–25 minutes to crisp the bread. Remove from the oven and set aside to cool.

3 Increase oven temperature to 350°F. Place prepared vegetables on a baking sheet, drizzle with 1 tablespoon olive oil, and season with salt and 1/8 teaspoon pepper. Roast in oven 15 minutes, turning halfway through cooking. Remove from oven and set aside.

4 While vegetables are roasting, prepare the vinaigrette by combining ⅓ cup olive oil, balsamic vinegar, mustard, and remaining black pepper in a liquid measuring cup. Whisk the ingredients together.

5 In a large mixing bowl, combine the bread cubes, arugula, roasted vegetables, and half of the balsamic vinaigrette. Toss to combine. You do not want to oversaturate the bread cubes, but they should soften a bit. Cover the bowl and allow salad to sit in the fridge 1 hour to "soak."

6 Add remaining dressing, mozzarella, and basil prior to serving. Enjoy within 24 hours.

Zucchini is one of my favorite summer vegetables because of its versatility, and this recipe is "no-cook," so it's perfect for summertime. While I wouldn't consider this a spicy dish, the chili garlic sauce will provide a little heat. This recipe is a good source of potassium with the zucchini, chickpeas, and Parmesan cheese. You could use a spiralizer to turn the zucchini into "zoodles" rather than ribbons. This recipe tastes great no matter how the zucchini is prepared!

Sleep-promoting ingredients	zucchini, chickpeas, cheese
Serves	2
Prep time	15 minutes
Cook time	N/A

Per Serving	
Calories	220
Fat	10 g
Protein	9 g
Sodium	270 mg
Fiber	7 g
Carbohydrates	27 g
Sugar	8 g

Zucchini Ribbons with Chickpeas and Olive Oil

1 tablespoon extra-virgin olive oil
1 teaspoon chili garlic sauce
2 medium zucchini
1 cup canned chickpeas, rinsed
¼ cup thinly sliced red onion
1 tablespoon grated Parmesan cheese
2 teaspoons lemon juice
⅛ teaspoon black pepper

1 In a small bowl, whisk together the olive oil and chili garlic sauce. Set aside.

2 Cut the top and bottom off of the zucchini. Using a vegetable peeler or a mandoline, slice the zucchini lengthwise into thin ribbons. Place ribbons in a medium bowl.

3 Add the chickpeas, red onion, Parmesan cheese, lemon juice, and pepper to the zucchini ribbons. Pour the chili oil over the mixture and mix together until everything is coated.

4 Serve immediately or keep refrigerated up to 24 hours.

Berry Coconut Smoothie Bowl

½ medium frozen zucchini, peeled and sliced
1 small frozen banana, sliced
4 fluid ounces light coconut milk
1 tablespoon fresh lime juice
1 teaspoon chia seeds

Toppings
¼ cup sliced strawberries
2 tablespoons fresh blueberries

1 Combine all ingredients except for toppings in a blender until smooth.

2 Pour into a bowl and top with strawberries and blueberries.

There's a hidden vegetable in this smoothie bowl that works well as breakfast or as a snack. Peeled frozen zucchini adds extra fiber and nutrients, plus it gives the smoothie bowl a nice creamy texture. This Berry Coconut Smoothie Bowl has a wonderful tropical flavor, so you can temporarily escape to the tropics no matter where you are.

Sleep-promoting ingredients	zucchini, banana, strawberries
Serves	1
Prep time	5 minutes
Cook time	N/A

Per Serving	
Calories	230
Fat	8 g
Protein	4 g
Sodium	65 mg
Fiber	7 g
Carbohydrates	41 g
Sugar	21 g

Get a good dose of omega-3 fatty acids with this simple recipe. Since the salmon is wrapped up inside foil packs with a marinade, it cooks to perfection. No more dry, overcooked fish! The other great part about this recipe is the minimal cleanup... always a bonus!

Sleep-promoting ingredients	cauliflower, salmon
Serves	4
Prep time	10 minutes
Cook time	19 minutes

Per Serving	
Calories	300
Fat	16 g
Protein	28 g
Sodium	105 mg
Fiber	5 g
Carbohydrates	16 g
Sugar	4 g

Sheet Pan Salmon and Vegetables

1 (12-ounce) package broccoli and cauliflower florets
1 (15-ounce) package diced butternut squash
3 tablespoons extra-virgin olive oil
1 tablespoon salt-free garlic and herb seasoning
4 (4-ounce) wild Alaskan salmon fillets
1 tablespoon Sprouts Organic Coconut Mango dressing, divided

1 Preheat oven to 425°F and line a large baking sheet with aluminum foil.

2 Make sure the broccoli and cauliflower florets are bite-sized pieces, then add to a large mixing bowl with the butternut squash. Add the olive oil and toss to coat vegetables. Pour the vegetables onto the baking sheet and sprinkle with the seasoning.

3 Place baking sheet on the middle rack in the oven and roast 5 minutes.

4 While the vegetables are roasting, tear off four sheets of aluminum foil large enough to wrap up each salmon fillet. Place each fillet on a piece of foil, skin side down, and pour 1 teaspoon of the dressing over each piece of salmon. Fold up the edges of the foil over the salmon to create a packet.

5 Remove baking sheet from oven and use a spatula to move the vegetables to one side of the sheet, making room for the salmon foil packets. Place sheet back in oven and roast 10–12 minutes.

6 To make sure the salmon is cooked through, carefully open one of the foil packets and use a fork to see if the fish is flaky. If it does not easily flake with the fork, place back in the oven 1–2 minutes.

7 Once the salmon is cooked through, use a spatula to carefully remove the salmon from the foil packet. It should easily release from the skin. Discard the foil.

8 Serve each salmon fillet with the roasted vegetables.

Tacos, with all of the toppings, are a great way to get in extra veggies at meal times. Cotija cheese can be found in most grocery stores in the specialty cheese section, usually near the deli case. It's a dense and crumbly cheese that has a bit of saltiness to it—perfect for these salmon tacos.

Sleep-promoting ingredients	salmon, avocado, tomato, cheese
Serves	4
Prep time	15 minutes
Cook time	21 minutes

Per Serving	
Calories	420
Fat	18 g
Protein	31 g
Sodium	470 mg
Fiber	2 g
Carbohydrates	37 g
Sugar	3 g

Blackened Salmon Tacos

2 ears corn, husks and silks removed
1 tablespoon paprika
1 teaspoon cayenne pepper
½ teaspoon salt, divided
1 (1-pound) wild Alaskan salmon fillet
2 teaspoons canola oil
5 fresh lime wedges
1 small ripe avocado, peeled and pitted
1 small Roma tomato, diced
2 tablespoons chopped cilantro leaves and stems
1 green onion, sliced thin, white and green parts separated
16 (5") corn tortillas
4 tablespoons Cotija cheese

1 Preheat oven broiler to 500°F and position top rack about 4" from the heat source.

2 Place corn on an aluminum foil–lined baking sheet and broil 10 minutes or until corn is slightly charred on all sides. Remove from oven and let cool. Remove corn from the cob.

3 Combine the paprika, cayenne pepper, and ¼ teaspoon salt in a small bowl. Pour spices onto a large plate. Place the flesh side of the salmon fillet into the spices, coating it well.

4 Heat a large cast-iron skillet over medium heat with the canola oil. Once the oil is hot, carefully place the salmon fillet into the skillet, flesh side down. Cook 2–3 minutes and then carefully flip salmon onto skin side and cook additional 6–8 minutes or until salmon can easily be flaked with a fork.

5 Place salmon on a large plate, squeeze one of the lime wedges over top, and allow to cool slightly before flaking the salmon into small pieces and removing the skin.

6 Meanwhile, make a salsa by mashing the avocado in a medium bowl. Add the tomato, cilantro, the white parts of the green onion, and remaining ¼ teaspoon salt and mix well.

7 For each taco use two corn tortillas to prevent them from breaking. Add the charred corn, salmon, avocado salsa, sliced green onion, and Cotija cheese. Squeeze lime wedge over the taco.

Lightly dressed and served cold, this salad is colorful and packed with fiber, vitamin A, vitamin C, and healthy fats. It's also lower in calories compared to mayonnaise-based potato salads. Sweet potatoes are a complex carbohydrate, meaning they are slowly digested and help prevent blood sugar spikes.

Sleep-promoting ingredients	sweet potato, avocado, yogurt
Serves	8
Prep time	20 minutes
Cook time	35 minutes

Per Serving	
Calories	180
Fat	7 g
Protein	6 g
Sodium	180 mg
Fiber	8 g
Carbohydrates	25 g
Sugar	5 g

Sweet Potato Fiesta Salad

3 medium sweet potatoes
2 tablespoons coconut oil
1 teaspoon chili powder
1 (15-ounce) can black beans, drained and rinsed
1 cup frozen corn kernels, thawed at room temperature
1 cup diced red bell pepper
2 green onions, sliced
1 large avocado, peeled, pitted, and diced
2 tablespoons cilantro leaves, roughly chopped

Cumin-Lime Dressing
¼ cup plain Greek yogurt
1 teaspoon lime juice
½ teaspoon ground cumin
¼ teaspoon salt

1 Preheat oven to 375°F.

2 Cut sweet potatoes into quarters. Place on baking sheet and coat in coconut oil and chili powder. Bake 23–25 minutes or until easily pierced with a fork.

3 Allow sweet potatoes to cool completely, then place in a large mixing bowl. Add all remaining ingredients to the sweet potatoes except for the Cumin-Lime Dressing.

4 In a small bowl, whisk together dressing ingredients. Pour over salad and mix well to coat. Keep refrigerated until ready to serve.

Loaded Southwest Sweet Potatoes

1 large sweet potato
⅛ teaspoon cayenne pepper
¼ cup shredded Mexican cheese
⅓ cup canned black beans, drained and rinsed well
¼ medium avocado, peeled, pitted, and sliced
1 tablespoon salsa
1 tablespoon cilantro

1 Preheat oven to 400°F. Line a baking sheet with aluminum foil.

2 Pierce the sweet potato several times with a knife and place on baking sheet. Bake 45–60 minutes or until you can easily pierce the sweet potato with a fork through the center.

3 Allow the sweet potato to cool slightly before cutting in half. Sprinkle cayenne pepper over the sweet potato, then top with cheese, beans, avocado, salsa, and cilantro.

We often think of loaded sweet potatoes as being smothered in marshmallows, brown sugar, and butter. While that version can be tasty, sweet potatoes are also delicious—and more nutritious—when topped with savory ingredients like black beans, avocado, and salsa. This meal is not only very filling, but also budget-friendly! The total cost for one serving comes in at under $1.50.

Sleep-promoting ingredients	sweet potato, cheese, avocado, tomato
Serves	1
Prep time	5 minutes
Cook time	45–60 minutes

Per Serving	
Calories	420
Fat	16 g
Protein	16 g
Sodium	390 mg
Fiber	15 g
Carbohydrates	57 g
Sugar	13 g

Here's a healthier, vegetarian twist on the classic patty melt. The trick to preparing good tofu is to drain it well and slice or cut it into small enough pieces that it loses the "jiggle."

Sleep-promoting ingredients	tofu, whole-grain bread, cheese
Serves	2
Prep time	10 minutes
Cook time	22 minutes

Per Serving	
Calories	410
Fat	22 g
Protein	24 g
Sodium	440 mg
Fiber	1 g
Carbohydrates	30 g
Sugar	4 g

Tofu Patty Melt

7 ounces extra-firm tofu, drained and pressed to remove liquid
1 tablespoon coconut oil
⅛ teaspoon garlic powder
⅛ teaspoon smoked paprika
⅓ cup sliced baby portobello mushrooms
¼ medium white onion, peeled and sliced thin
¼ medium green bell pepper, seeded and sliced thin
4 slices whole-wheat bread
2 slices Muenster cheese

1 Place tofu block on a cutting board and slice four (½"-thick) slices.

2 Heat oil in a large skillet over medium-high heat. Add tofu slices, season with garlic powder and paprika, and cook 5 minutes. Flip tofu slices and cook 2 more minutes. Once crispy, remove tofu and set aside.

3 Sauté vegetables in same skillet over medium heat until tender, about 4–5 minutes. Remove and set aside.

4 Assemble the sandwiches using bread, cheese slices, crispy tofu, and sautéed vegetables. Heat a griddle pan or griddle appliance over medium heat. Spray griddle with cooking spray before placing sandwich on griddle. Grill each side of the sandwich until crispy and cheese is melted, about 5 minutes on each side. Serve immediately.

Chocolate Cherry Smoothie

1 cup soy milk
1 cup frozen tart cherries
¼ cup silken tofu
2 tablespoons cocoa powder
4 pitted dates, roughly chopped

1 Combine all ingredients in a blender.

2 Process until smooth, about 20 seconds.

To press tofu, stack two paper towels on a plate or cutting board. Place the tofu on top. Add two more paper towels and then place a plate on top of the tofu block to press it. Let this sit 1–2 minutes. If the tofu is still saturated, replace the paper towels and repeat the process.

Chocolate and cherries were just meant to be together. This deliciously creamy smoothie is naturally sweetened with cherries and dates, and it makes a great post-workout snack. Silken tofu works well in smoothies, providing a creamy texture and a source of protein to help keep you feeling satisfied and to minimize a spike in blood sugar levels. You can use 1% or 2% milk instead of soy milk, if you prefer.

Sleep-promoting ingredients	milk, tart cherries, tofu, dates
Serves	2
Prep time	5 minutes
Cook time	N/A

Per Serving	
Calories	180
Fat	3.5 g
Protein	7 g
Sodium	65 mg
Fiber	5 g
Carbohydrates	33 g
Sugar	23 g

The key to making spring rolls is having all of your ingredients prepped ahead of time and cut into similar sizes. The rice paper sheets might be a bit tricky to work with at first, but after a couple, you'll get the hang of it! Rice paper sheets can be found in most grocery stores in the international section or in Asian supermarkets.

Sleep-promoting ingredients	tofu, cucumber, avocado
Serves	4
Prep time	10 minutes
Cook time	N/A

Per Serving	
Calories	430
Fat	26 g
Protein	17 g
Sodium	160 mg
Fiber	5 g
Carbohydrates	36 g
Sugar	7 g

Tofu Spring Rolls with Carrot Ginger Sauce

Carrot Ginger Sauce
1 cup shredded carrots
¼ cup plus 1 tablespoon sesame oil
2 tablespoons water
1 tablespoon rice vinegar
1 tablespoon creamy peanut butter
1 tablespoon 100 percent pure maple syrup
1 tablespoon tamari or low-sodium soy sauce
1" piece fresh ginger, skin removed

Tofu Spring Rolls
14 ounces extra-firm tofu, drained and pressed to remove liquid
12 rice paper sheets
1 small head Boston lettuce
1 medium cucumber, cut into thin strips
½ medium red bell pepper, seeded and cut into thin strips
1 medium avocado, peeled, pitted, and sliced into thin strips
1 tablespoon sriracha
4 tablespoons fresh cilantro leaves
2 cups sunflower sprouts, rinsed and patted dry

1 Prepare Carrot Ginger Sauce: Combine all sauce ingredients in a blender or small food processor and process until smooth, about 30 seconds. Place into a small bowl and refrigerate until ready to use.

2 Prepare Tofu Spring Rolls: Cut the tofu block in half and then cut each piece in half again. Cut each piece into thin strips (you will need twenty-four thin strips total).

3 Before assembling spring rolls, place all prepared ingredients on a cutting board for easy assembly and have a large plate or cutting board to roll spring rolls.

4 Prepare rice paper wrappers according to package directions. Place soaked wrapper on plate and start by placing lettuce leaf on wrapper, followed by two pieces each of tofu, cucumber, red bell pepper, and avocado. Add a thin line of sriracha and then top with cilantro and sunflower sprouts.

5 Roll the spring roll by folding the portion of the wrapper closest to you over the ingredients, being sure to tuck in all the ingredients before folding the edges over and continuing to roll up until sealed.

6 Place spring rolls on a plate and serve with prepared Carrot Ginger Sauce. Keep stored in an airtight container up to 48 hours in the refrigerator.

No cooking is required for this flavorful superfood salad! Even those who don't usually like cauliflower can enjoy this recipe since the cauliflower is chopped into such small pieces using a food processor. This salad is loaded with antioxidants from the cauliflower, kale, cranberries, and red onion, and it is naturally vegan and gluten-free.

Sleep-promoting ingredients	cauliflower, chickpeas, pumpkin seeds
Serves	6
Prep time	15 minutes
Cook time	N/A

Per Serving	
Calories	240
Fat	8 g
Protein	7 g
Sodium	210 mg
Fiber	7 g
Carbohydrates	38 g
Sugar	20 g

Cauliflower Cranberry Superfood Salad

1 small head cauliflower (about 3½ cups florets)
1 cup finely chopped Tuscan kale
¾ cup dried cranberries, chopped
½ cup finely diced red onion
1 (15-ounce) can chickpeas, drained and rinsed
3 tablespoons raw pumpkin seeds
2 tablespoons olive oil
2 tablespoons balsamic vinegar
1 clove garlic, peeled and minced
⅛ teaspoon salt
⅛ teaspoon black pepper

1 Place the cauliflower florets in the bowl of a food processor, filling it ¾ full. Use the pulse button to process the cauliflower until it is broken down into rice-sized pieces. Using a spatula, remove cauliflower from food processor and place in a large mixing bowl.

2 Add the kale, cranberries, red onion, chickpeas, and pumpkin seeds to the cauliflower. Mix well.

3 In a small bowl, whisk together the olive oil, balsamic vinegar, and garlic. Pour over the cauliflower salad and mix well.

4 Season the salad with salt and pepper. Serve chilled. Salad will keep up to three days in the refrigerator.

Veggie-Stuffed Zucchini

1 medium zucchini
½ tablespoon olive oil, divided
½ teaspoon fresh minced garlic
¼ cup finely diced red onion
½ cup chopped mushrooms
1 cup finely chopped cauliflower
1 cup finely chopped kale
½ teaspoon salt-free garlic and herb seasoning
⅛ teaspoon salt
⅛ teaspoon black pepper
2 tablespoons grated Parmesan cheese

1 Preheat oven to 350°F.

2 Cut zucchini in half lengthwise and scoop out inner flesh to make a well for filling. Place zucchini halves on a baking sheet and lightly drizzle with half of the olive oil. Bake 15 minutes.

3 While the zucchini is in the oven, heat remaining olive oil in a medium skillet over medium heat for 1 minute. Add garlic, red onion, and mushrooms. Sauté 3 minutes.

4 Add cauliflower to the skillet and cook an additional 5 minutes. Add kale, seasoning, salt, and pepper, stirring to combine.

5 Spoon vegetable mixture into the zucchini halves and top with Parmesan cheese. Bake 13–15 minutes or until zucchini is tender and cheese is melted.

Similar to stuffed peppers or stuffed mushrooms, zucchini filled with vegetables makes for a fiber-rich meal. This recipe has less than 20 grams of carbohydrates and can easily be doubled to make more servings. You could also serve this alongside seared salmon or chicken for additional protein.

Sleep-promoting ingredients	zucchini, cauliflower
Serves	1
Prep time	15 minutes
Cook time	38 minutes

Per Serving	
Calories	200
Fat	11 g
Protein	9 g
Sodium	530 mg
Fiber	6 g
Carbohydrates	20 g
Sugar	10 g

Three-Day Meal Plan

This meal plan is a general guide to including more of the sleep-promoting foods listed in this book into your daily routine. Feel free to swap out recipes or certain foods with others included in the book and tweak them to meet your needs. Remember, everyone is different in their nutritional needs and average daily calorie needs, so if you are looking for tailored nutrition guidance, visit with a registered dietitian. This meal plan will be a good starting point to get you back to consistently good sleep and energy-filled days.

DAY 1

Calories	1,692
Fat	62 g
Protein	82 g
Sodium	1,703 mg
Fiber	36 g
Carbohydrates	220 g

Breakfast	Egg on Avocado Toast with Salsa
	½ cup cantaloupe cubes
	4 fluid ounces 1% milk
	4 fluid ounces tart cherry juice
Morning Snack	1 serving Chocolate Cherry Smoothie with 20 baby carrots
Lunch	Cucumber Tartine with 1 cup diced watermelon
	8 fluid ounces water
Afternoon Snack	Banana and Walnut Trail Mix
	6 fluid ounces coconut water
Dinner	1 serving Blackened Salmon Tacos
	⅓ cup brown rice
	1 cup broccoli
	1 cup cauliflower
	8 fluid ounces water
Evening Snack	8 fluid ounces chamomile tea
	5 whole-wheat crackers
	1 tablespoon cashew butter

DAY 2

Calories	1,801
Fat	71 g
Protein	101 g
Sodium	841 mg
Fiber	31 g
Carbohydrates	204 g

Breakfast	Chocolate Cherry Oatmeal
	4 fluid ounces 1% milk
	8 fluid ounces water
Morning Snack	1 medium banana
	12 almonds
	8 fluid ounces unsweetened iced green tea
Lunch	1 serving Tofu Spring Rolls with Carrot Ginger Sauce
	1 cup cherries
	½ cup edamame
	8 fluid ounces water
Dinner	1 serving Roasted Summer Vegetable Panzanella
	3 ounces cooked top sirloin steak
	½ cup cooked quinoa
	8 fluid ounces water
Evening Snack	1 cup peppermint herbal tea
	½ cup strawberries
	½ cup cottage cheese

DAY 3

Calories	1,687
Fat	52 g
Protein	129 g
Sodium	1,352 mg
Fiber	33 g
Carbohydrates	182 g

Breakfast	1 serving Greek Quinoa Breakfast Bowl
	4 fluid ounces tart cherry juice
Morning Snack	¾ cup plain Greek nonfat yogurt with ⅓ cup blueberries
	¼ cup strawberries
	8 fluid ounces water
Lunch	1 serving Zesty Tuna Lettuce Wraps
	1 large apple
	8 fluid ounces water
Afternoon Snack	2 pieces Chocolate Banana Oat Bites
	6 fluid ounces coconut water
Dinner	1 serving Zucchini Ribbons with Chickpeas and Olive Oil
	4 ounces roasted turkey breast
	8 fluid ounces water
Evening Snack	10 small celery stalks
	3 tablespoons hummus
	4 fluid ounces 1% milk

Best Bedtime Snacks

Choosing the right foods to snack on before bedtime is an important part of a healthy sleep routine. If you're consistently snacking on foods that can interfere with sleep, as listed in Chapter 2, or overconsuming calories before bed, a sleepless night may lie ahead. Instead, opt for one of these bedtime snack combinations, or create your own snack combo from foods listed in Chapter 3. Doing so will help you get a balance of complex carbohydrates and protein to help keep blood sugar levels stabilized throughout the night and to keep you feeling satisfied, without causing stomach discomfort. In regard to drinking fluids before bed, find what works best for you in terms of timing to prevent having to get up in the middle of the night to use the bathroom. Keep in mind that no matter what time of day you eat snacks, they should be chosen wisely for the nutrients they provide your body.

Here are some bedtime snack ideas:

- Cottage cheese with fruit such as cherries or strawberries
- Banana with peanut butter or almonds
- Whole-wheat toast with nut butter and sliced banana
- Celery with hummus or light herbed cream cheese
- Homemade popcorn with Parmesan cheese
- Chamomile tea with a few whole-wheat crackers and sliced white cheddar cheese
- Chocolate-dipped strawberries (if not sensitive to caffeine content of dark chocolate)
- Greek yogurt with almonds
- Glass of milk with a small banana

CHAPTER 5

Food and Sleep Log

You've learned a lot about how food choices, daily activities, and the surrounding environment can impact your sleep, both positively and negatively. Now that you're armed with the knowledge about how to improve your sleep, it will be helpful to have a way to keep track of the changes you've made so you can determine what's working and what isn't working for you.

Logging your food can help you discover patterns you may not necessarily pick up on until you take the time to write them down. Having a log to refer back to may help you connect the dots between choices you make during the day and how they affect you at night. Personally, it took me quite some time to recognize that red wine in the evening, even with meals, was guaranteed to have me tossing and turning that very night. Once I decided to pay attention and connect those dots, it was easy to zero in on the problem and make appropriate changes.

You can select three (or however many you feel apply to you!) of the following areas to focus on to help improve sleep. If you think there are improvements you can make in each of these areas, I'd suggest starting off with a few simple changes that you can easily implement. Let's face it: change can be hard, but when you set small, attainable, realistic goals for yourself, it's much easier to stick with them. Here's an example:

For the next week, I will not drink any caffeinated beverages after noon.

This is a very specific goal that has a time frame (one week) so that you can hold yourself accountable. If you see positive effects from the changes you decide to make, then of course carry on with them! If you don't notice any changes in your sleep patterns, it will be important to consider what other factors may be interfering with sleep. Another reason why this Food and Sleep Log is so important!

Top Factors to Focus On to Improve Sleep

- Diet
- Exercise
- Stress management
- Activities before bed
- Caffeine intake in the afternoon
- Alcohol intake in the evening
- Noise disturbances

Now, write three sleep-related changes you plan to implement this month.

1. _____

_____

_____

2. _____

_____

_____

3. _____

_____

_____

Daily Log Entry

Here are some things you should include in your daily entry:

Time you went to bed:

_____

Time you woke up:

_____

Did you wake up during the night?

_____

Did you consume caffeine or alcohol? If yes, what time?

_____

Did you have any sleep-promoting foods today? If yes, list them:

_____

What activities were you doing 30 minutes before bed?
(watching TV, looking at your phone, reading a book, and so on)

_____

Any particularly stressful topics on your mind?

_____

Good Sleep Checklist

Week of:

_____

During the Day Activities

◯ Eat a variety of foods listed in Chapter 3 throughout the day
◯ Exercise for 30 minutes (at least 3–4 hours before going to bed)
◯ Stay adequately hydrated throughout the day
◯ Avoid excessive intake of refined sugar during the day
◯ Avoid high-fat meals, alcohol, caffeine, and big meals at least 3–4 hours before bed

Before Bed Activities

◯ Turn off electronics 1 hour before bed
◯ Turn down thermostat to keep room cooler while sleeping
◯ Try meditation techniques and use an app to help with breathing exercises
◯ Try using aromatherapy, such as lavender oil, to create a calming environment
◯ Write in a journal or read a book
◯ Use a sound machine or white noise app to limit sound interruptions

APPENDIX B

References

Abdollahnejad, F., M. Mosaddegh, M. Kamalinejad, J. Mirnajafi-Zadeh, F. Najafi, and M. Faizi. "Investigation of Sedative and Hypnotic Effects of Amygdalus communis L. Extract: Behavioral Assessments and EEG Studies on Rat." *Journal of Natural Medicines* 70, no. 2 (April 2016): 190–197. https://doi.org/10.1007/s11418-015-0958-9.

AddictionCenter.com. "Addiction to Ambien." www.addictioncenter.com/sleeping-pills/ambien/ (accessed September 8, 2018).

AgHires. "The U.S. Produces Over 70% of the World's Mint." (2017) https://aghires.com/u-s-produces-70-worlds-mint/ (accessed September 13, 2018).

Agricultural Marketing Resource Center. "Cauliflower." (2018) www.agmrc.org/commodities-products/vegetables/cauliflower (accessed September 23, 2018).

Agricultural Marketing Resource Center. "Celery." (2018) www.agmrc.org/commodities-products/vegetables/celery-profile (accessed January 20, 2019).

Agricultural Marketing Resource Center. "Chickpeas." (2018) www.agmrc.org/commodities-products/vegetables/chickpeas (accessed October 21, 2018).

Agricultural Marketing Resource Center. "Citrus." (2015) www.agmrc.org/commodities-products/fruits/citrus/citrus-profile (accessed January 21, 2019).

Agricultural Marketing Resource Center. "Melons." (2018) www.agmrc.org/commodities-products/vegetables/melons (accessed September 17, 2018).

Agricultural Marketing Resource Center. "Squash." (2018) www.agmrc.org/commodities-products/vegetables/squash (accessed October 26, 2018).

Agricultural Marketing Resource Center. "Sweet Potatoes." (2018) www.agmrc .org/commodities-products/vegetables/sweet-potatoes (accessed October 25, 2018).

Almond Board of California. "Health and Nutrition." (2018) www.almonds.com/ consumers/health-and-nutrition (accessed September 24, 2018).

American Dairy Association Northeast. "Cheese & Nutrition Brochure." (2017) www.americandairy.com/_resources/documents/cheese-brochure.pdf (accessed January 25, 2019).

American Pistachio Growers. "Nutrition Power." https://americanpistachios .org/nutrition-and-health/nutrition-power (accessed January 20, 2019).

Ancient Grains. "Quinoa History and Origin." www.ancientgrains.com/ quinoa-history-and-origin/ (accessed October 28, 2018).

Anxiety and Depression Association of America. "Helpful Guide to Different Therapy Options." https://adaa.org/finding-help/treatment/therapy (accessed September 9, 2018).

Avey, T. PBS. "Uncover the History of Pasta." (2012) www.pbs.org/food/ the-history-kitchen/uncover-the-history-of-pasta/ (accessed September 24, 2018).

Basu, T. *The Atlantic*. "The Secret Life of String Cheese." (2014) www.the atlantic.com/technology/archive/2014/11/the-secret-life-of-string-cheese/ 383001/ (accessed October 29, 2018).

BBC. "Pumpkin's Surprising Origin." www.bbc.com/travel/story/20151027-pumpkins-surprising-origin (accessed January 21, 2019).

Beef. It's What's for Dinner. "Top Sirloin Steak." (2018) www.beefitswhatsfor dinner.com/cuts/cut/2775/top-sirloin-steak (accessed October 29, 2018).

Burton, J. *World Atlas*. "The World Leaders in Coconut Production." (2018) www.worldatlas.com/articles/the-world-leaders-in-coconut-production.html (accessed September 20, 2018).

Cafasso, J. Healthline. "Valerian Root Dosage for Anxiety and Sleep." (2016) www.healthline.com/health/food-nutrition/valerian-root (accessed October 29, 2018).

California Avocados. "The History of California Avocados." (2018) www
.californiaavocado.com/avocado101/the-california-difference/avocado-history
(accessed October 20, 2018).

California Dried Plums. "Bone Health." (2018) www.californiadriedplums.org/
nutrition/bone-health (accessed October 28, 2018).

California Strawberries. "What's in a Strawberry?" (2018) www.california
strawberries.com/welcome/8-a-day/whats-in-a-strawberry/ (accessed
September 27, 2018).

California Walnuts. "History." https://walnuts.org/about-walnuts/history/
(accessed October 26, 2018).

Centers for Disease Control and Prevention. "1 in 3 Adults Don't Get Enough
Sleep." (2016) www.cdc.gov/media/releases/2016/p0215-enough-sleep.html
(accessed September 8, 2018).

Centers for Disease Control and Prevention. "Drowsy Driving: Asleep at
the Wheel." www.cdc.gov/features/dsdrowsydriving/index.html (accessed
September 9, 2018).

Chagas, M.H.N., J.A.S. Crippa, A.W. Zuardi, J.E.C. Hallak, J.P. Machado-de-
Sousa, C. Hirotsu, L. Maia, S. Tufik, and M.L. Andersen. "Effects of Acute
Systemic Administration of Cannabidiol on Sleep-Wake Cycle in Rats." *Journal
of Psychopharmacology* 27, no. 3 (January 2013): 312–316. www.researchgate
.net/publication/235366318_Effects_of_acute_systemic_administration_of_
cannabidiol_on_sleep-wake_cycle_in_rats.

Chang, S.M., and C.H. Chen. "Effects of an Intervention with Drinking
Chamomile Tea on Sleep Quality and Depression in Sleep Disturbed Postnatal
Women: A Randomized Controlled Trial." *Journal of Advanced Nursing* 72, no.
2 (October 2015): 306–15. https://doi.org/10.1111/jan.12836.

Chollet, D., P. Franken, Y. Raffin, J.G. Henrotte, J. Widmer, A. Malafosse, and
M. Tafti. "Magnesium Involvement in Sleep: Genetic and Nutritional Models."
Behavior Genetics 31, no. 5 (September 2001): 413–425. PMID: 11777170.

Cleveland Clinic. "Omega-3 Fatty Acids." (2017) https://my.clevelandclinic.org/
health/articles/17290-omega-3-fatty-acids/how-much-omega-3-do-i-need
(accessed October 10, 2018).

Cui, Y., K. Niu, C. Huang, H. Momma, L. Guan, Y. Kobayashi, H. Guo, M. Chujo, A. Otomo, and R. Nagatomi. "Relationship Between Daily Isoflavone Intake and Sleep in Japanese Adults: A Cross-Sectional Study." *Nutrition Journal* 14, no. 1 (December 2015): 127. https://doi.org/10.1186/s12937-015-0117-x.

Dairy Goodness. "The History of Yogurt." www.dairygoodness.ca/yogurt/the-history-of-yogurt (accessed September 30, 2018).

Dietary Guidelines 2015–2020. "Chapter 2: Shifts Needed to Align with Healthy Eating Patterns." (2015) https://health.gov/dietaryguidelines/2015/guidelines/chapter-2/a-closer-look-at-current-intakes-and-recommended-shifts/ (accessed September 28, 2018).

Dietitians of Canada. "Food Sources of Vitamin B6." www.dietitians.ca/getattachment/ea1272c8-602f-4586-8ffb-d7b4a2535634/FACTSHEET-Food-Sources-of-Vitamin-B6.pdf.aspx (accessed January 19, 2019).

Drews, K., A. Seremak-Mrozikiewicz, E. Puk, A. Kaluba-Skotarczak, M. Malec, and A. Kazikowska. "Efficacy of Standardized Isoflavones Extract (Soyfem) (52–104 mg/24h) in Moderate and Medium-Severe Climacteric Syndrome." *Ginekologia Polska* 78, no. 4 (April 2007): 307–311. PMID: 17621994.

Egg Nutrition Center. "Cardiometabolic Health." www.eggnutritioncenter.org/topics/cardiometabolic-health (accessed October 22, 2018).

Egg Nutrition Center. "Eggs 101 – Egg FAQ's." www.eggnutritioncenter.org/egg-facts/ (accessed October 22, 2018).

Encyclopedia Britannica. "Salmon." www.britannica.com/animal/salmon (accessed October 24, 2018).

Fruits and Veggies—More Matters. "Green Soybeans (Edamame): Nutrition. Selection. Storage." www.fruitsandveggiesmorematters.org/green-soybeans-edamame-nutrition-selection-storage (accessed October 28, 2018).

Fruits and Veggies—More Matters. "Medjool Dates: Nutrition. Selection. Storage." www.fruitsandveggiesmorematters.org/medjool-dates-nutrition-selection-storage (accessed October 27, 2018).

Goyal, A., V. Sharma, N. Upadhyay, S. Gill, and M. Sihag. "Flax and Flaxseed Oil: An Ancient Medicine & Modern Functional Food." *Journal of Food Science and Technology* 51, no. 9 (September 2014): 1,633–1,653. https://doi.org/10.1007%2Fs13197-013-1247-9.

Grains & Legumes Nutrition Council. "Legumes and Nutrition." www.glnc.org.au/legumes-2/legumes-and-nutrition/ (accessed January 19, 2019).

Hamilton, J. NPR. "Apps Can Cut Blue Light from Devices, but Do They Help You Sleep?" (2017) www.npr.org/sections/health-shots/2017/11/27/561740031/apps-can-cut-blue-light-from-devices-but-do-they-help-you-sleep (accessed September 9, 2018).

Harvard Health Publishing. "Key Minerals to Help Control Blood Pressure." (2014) www.health.harvard.edu/heart-health/key-minerals-to-help-control-blood-pressure (accessed September 24, 2018).

Healthline. "Is Phosphoric Acid Bad for Me?" www.healthline.com/health/food-nutrition/is-phosphoric-acid-bad-for-me#1 (accessed January 20, 2019).

Herbst, S.T., and R. Herbst. *Food Lover's Companion: 4th Edition.* (Hauppauge, NY: Barron's Educational Series, Inc., 2007).

History. "A Brief History of Bread." (2012) www.history.com/news/a-brief-history-of-bread (accessed September 24, 2018).

Hurst, Y., and H. Fukuda. "Effects of Changes in Eating Speed on Obesity in Patients with Diabetes: A Secondary Analysis of Longitudinal Health Check-Up Data." *BMJ Open* 8, no. 1 (February 2018): e019589. https://doi.org/10.1136/bmjopen-2017-019589.

Jenkins, T.A., J.C.D. Nguyen, K.E. Polglaze, and P.P. Bertrand. "Influence of Tryptophan and Serotonin on Mood and Cognition with a Possible Role of the Gut-Brain Axis." *Nutrients* 8, no. 1 (January 2016): 56. https://doi.org/10.3390/nu8010056.

Knutson, K.L., A.M. Ryden, B.A. Mander, and E. Van Cauter. "Role of Sleep Duration and Quality in the Risk and Severity of Type 2 Diabetes Mellitus." *Archives of Internal Medicine* 166, no. 16 (September 2006): 1,768–1,774. https://doi.org/10.1001/archinte.166.16.1768.

Kummer, C. *The Atlantic. The Rise of the Sardine*. (2007) www.theatlantic.com/magazine/archive/2007/07/the-rise-of-the-sardine/305976/ (accessed October 24, 2018).

Loprinzi, P.D., and B.J. Cardinal. "Association Between Objectively-Measured Physical Activity and Sleep, NHANES 2005–2006." *Mental Health and Physical Activity* 4, no. 2 (December 2011): 65–69. https://doi.org/10.1016/j.mhpa.2011.08.001.

Losso, J.N., J.W. Finley, N. Karki, A. Liu, A. Prudente, R. Tipton, Y. Yu, and F. Greenway. "Pilot Study of the Tart Cherry Juice for the Treatment of Insomnia and Investigation of Mechanisms." *American Journal of Therapeutics* 25, no. 2 (March/April 2018): 194–201. https://doi.org/10.1097/MJT.0000000000000584.

Malhorta, S., G. Sawhney, and P. Pandhi. Medscape. "The Therapeutic Potential of Melatonin: A Review of the Science." *Medscape General Medicine* 6, no. 2 (April 2004): 46. www.medscape.com/viewarticle/472385_1 (accessed September 28, 2018).

Mayo Clinic. "Caffeine Content for Coffee, Tea, Soda, and More." (2017) www.mayoclinic.org/healthy-lifestyle/nutrition-and-healthy-eating/in-depth/caffeine/art-20049372 (accessed August 15, 2018).

McHugh, T. Institute of Food Technologists. "How Tofu Is Processed." (2016) www.ift.org/food-technology/past-issues/2016/february/columns/processing-how-tofu-is-processed.aspx?page=viewall (accessed October 28, 2018).

Meng, X., Y. Li., S. Li, Y. Zhou, R.Y. Gan, D.P. Xu, and H.B. Li. "Dietary Sources and Bioactivities of Melatonin." *Nutrients* 9, no. 4 (April 2017): 367. https://doi.org/10.3390/nu9040367.

Monterey Bay Aquarium Seafood Watch. "Salmon Overview." (2018) www.seafoodwatch.org/seafood-recommendations/groups/salmon/overview (accessed October 24, 2018).

Montmorency US Tart Cherries. "Tart Cherries 101." www.choosecherries.com/tart-cherries-101/ (accessed August 15, 2018).

Murray, M.T., and J. Pizzorno. *The Encyclopedia of Natural Medicine: 3rd Edition*. (New York: Atria, 2012).

National Geographic. "Why Are Bananas So Cheap?" www.nationalgeographic .com/people-and-culture/food/the-plate/2016/08/bananas-are-so-cool/ (accessed January 19, 2019).

National Institutes of Health. "Valerian." https://ods.od.nih.gov/factsheets/ Valerian-HealthProfessional/#en1 (accessed January 23, 2019).

National Sleep Foundation. "Study: Physical Activity Impacts Overall Quality of Sleep." www.sleepfoundation.org/sleep-news/study-physical-activity-impacts-overall-quality-sleep (accessed January 22, 2019).

National Sunflower Association. "History of the Amazing Sunflower." www .sunflowernsa.com/all-about/history/ (accessed October 29, 2018).

National Turkey Federation. "Healthy Eating Made Easy." (2018) www.eatturkey .org/healthy-eating-made-easy/ (accessed October 10, 2018).

New World Encyclopedia. "Grapefruit." (2017) www.newworldencyclopedia .org/entry/Grapefruit (accessed October 27, 2018).

Newsday, E.M. "The Juicy History of the Orange in America." (2008) www.sun-sentinel.com/news/fl-xpm-2008-05-22-0805200422-story.html (accessed October 28, 2018).

Nielsen, F.H., L.K. Johnson, and H. Zeng. "Magnesium Supplementation Improves Indicators of Low Magnesium Status and Inflammatory Stress in Adults Older Than 51 Years with Poor Quality Sleep." *Magnesium Research* 23, no. 4 (December 2010): 158–68. https://pdfs.semanticscholar.org/2961/ 39514f1fde29604c5237ba19002a8042d155.pdf.

Nishiura, C., and H. Hashimoto. "A 4-Year Study of the Association Between Short Sleep Duration and Change in Body Mass Index in Japanese Male Workers." *Journal of Epidemiology* 20, no. 5 (August 2010): 385–390. https:// doi.org/10.2188/jea.JE20100019.

Patel, S.R., A. Malhotra, D.P. White, D.J. Gottlieb, and F.B. Hu. "Association Between Reduced Sleep and Weight Gain in Women." *American Journal of Epidemiology* 164, no. 10 (August 2006): 947–954. https://doi.org/10.1093/aje/ kwj280.

Planet Natural Research Center. "History of Tomatoes." www.planetnatural .com/tomato-gardening-guru/history/ (accessed October 29, 2018).

Reiter, R.J., L.C. Manchester, and D.X. Tan. "Melatonin in Walnuts: Influence on Levels of Melatonin and Total Antioxidant Capacity of Blood." *Nutrition* 21, no. 9 (September 2005): 920–924. https://doi.org/10.1016/j.nut.2005.02.005.

Reuters. "Americans Are Drinking a Daily Cup of Coffee at the Highest Level in Six Years: Survey." www.reuters.com/article/us-coffee-conference-survey/americans-are-drinking-a-daily-cup-of-coffee-at-the-highest-level-in-six-years-survey-idUSKCN1GT0KU (accessed January 19, 2019).

Rivlin, R.S. "Magnesium Deficiency and Alcohol Intake: Mechanisms, Clinical Significance and Possible Relation to Cancer Development (a Review)." *Journal of the American College of Nutrition* 13, no. 5 (October 1994): 416–423.

Sánchez, E., F. De Gioia, L.F. Kime, and J.K. Harper. PennState Extension. "Cucumber Production." (2015) https://extension.psu.edu/cucumber-production (accessed October 10, 2018).

ScienceDaily. "Sleep Loss Boosts Appetite, May Encourage Weight Gain." (2004) www.sciencedaily.com/releases/2004/12/041206210355.htm (accessed January 24, 2019).

Shokri-Kojori, E., et al. "β-Amyloid Accumulation in the Human Brain after One Night of Sleep Deprivation." *Proceedings of the National Academy of Sciences of the United States of America* 115, no. 17 (April 2018): 4483–4488. https://doi.org/10.1073/pnas.1721694115.

Shukla, S., and S. Gupta. "Apigenin: A Promising Molecule for Cancer Prevention." *Pharmaceutical Research* 27, no. 6 (March 2010): 962–978. https://doi.org/10.107/s11095-010-0089-7.

Shurtleff, W., and A. Aoyagi. Soy Info Center. "History of Tofu–Page 5." (2004) www.soyinfocenter.com/HSS/tofu5.php (accessed October 28, 2018).

Singh, O., Z. Khanam, N. Misra, and M.K. Srivastava. "Chamomile (*Matricaria chamomilla* L.): An Overview." *Pharmacognosy Review* 5, no. 9 (January 2011): 82–95. www.ncbi.nlm.nih.gov/pmc/articles/PMC3210003/.

Specialty Food Association. "US Quinoa Consumption Rises Dramatically." (2016) www.specialtyfood.com/news/article/us-quinoa-consumption-rises-dramatically/ (accessed October 28, 2018).

Stone, D. *National Geographic.* "The Miracle of the Modern Banana." (2016) www.nationalgeographic.com/people-and-culture/food/the-plate/2016/08/the-miracle-of-bananas/ (accessed September 15, 2018).

Taavoni, S., N. Ekbatani, M. Kashaniyan, and H. Haghani. "Effect of Valerian on Sleep Quality in Postmenopausal Women: A Randomized Placebo-Controlled Clinical Trial." *Menopause* 18, no. 9 (September 2011): 951–955. https://doi.org/10.1097/gme.0b013e31820e9acf.

Taheri, S. "The Link Between Short Sleep Duration and Obesity: We Should Recommend More Sleep to Prevent Obesity." *Archives of Disease in Childhood* 91, no. 11 (October 2006): 881–884. https://doi.org/10.1136/adc.2005.093013.

Teatulia. "What Is Chamomile?" www.teatulia.com/tea-varieties/what-is-chamomile.htm (accessed January 20, 2019).

The Beef Checkoff. "Beef & Health: A Fresh Look at Today's Beef." (2017) www.iabeef.org/Media/IABeef/Docs/beef_and_health_053116-01.pdf (accessed October 27, 2018).

The Incredible Egg. "The History of the Egg." www.incredibleegg.org/egg-nutrition/#history-of-the-egg (accessed October 22, 2018).

US Food and Drug Administration. "Eating Fish: What Pregnant Women and Parents Should Know." (2017) www.fda.gov/Food/ResourcesForYou/Consumers/ucm393070.htm (accessed October 28, 2018).

Vegetable Facts. "Spinach History—Origins of Different Types of Spinach." (2018) www.vegetablefacts.net/vegetable-history/spinach-history/ (accessed October 25, 2018).

Watermelon.org. "Health 101." (2018) www.watermelon.org/Nutrition/Health-101 (accessed October 16, 2018).

WebMD. "Valerian." www.webmd.com/vitamins/ai/ingredientmono-870/valerian (accessed October 29, 2018).

Whole Grains Council. "Barley—February Grain of the Month." https://wholegrainscouncil.org/whole-grains-101/grain-month-calendar/barley-%E2%80%93-february-grain-month (accessed January 20, 2019).

Whole Grains Council. "Whole Grains A to Z." https://wholegrainscouncil.org/whole-grains-101/whole-grains-z (accessed September 18, 2018).

Woolston, C. AARP. "Using Pills to Fall Asleep at Night?" www.aarp.org/health/drugs-supplements/info-07-2013/sleeping-pill-side-effects.html (accessed September 8, 2018).

Workman, D. World's Top Exports. "Barley Exports by Country." (2018) www.worldstopexports.com/barley-exports-by-country/ (accessed September 15, 2018).

Young, S. "How to Increase Serotonin in the Human Brain Without Drugs." *Journal of Psychiatry and Neuroscience* 32, no. 6 (November 2007): 394–399. PMID: 18043762.

Zhou, J., J.E. Kim, C.L.H. Armstrong, N. Chen, and W.W. Campbell. "Higher-Protein Diets Improve Indexes of Sleep in Energy-Restricted Overweight and Obese Adults: Results from 2 Randomized Controlled Trials." *The American Journal of Clinical Nutrition* 103, no. 3 (February 2016): 766–774. https:doi.org/10.3945/ajcn.115.124669.

Index

Note: Page numbers in *italics* indicate recipes.

Acidic foods, sleep and, 39–40
Almonds, 46–47, 156, 158–59
Aromatherapy, for sleep, 24–25
Avocados
    about: history of, 49; how and when
        to enjoy, 48–49; nutrition facts, 49;
        sleep and health benefits, 48
    Blackened Salmon Tacos, *172–73*
    Egg on Avocado Toast with Salsa, *152*
    other recipes with, *154–55, 161, 164–
        65, 174, 175, 178–79*

Bananas
    about: history of, 51; how and when to
        enjoy, 51; nutrition facts, 51; sleep
        and health benefits, 50
    Banana and Walnut Trail Mix, *157*
    Berry Coconut Smoothie Bowl, *169*
    Chocolate Banana Oat Bites, *158–59*
Barley, about, 52–53
Beans and other legumes
    about: chickpeas, 70–71; edamame,
        80–81; history of, 71, 81; how
        and when to enjoy, 70–71, 80–81;
        nutrition facts, 71, 81; sleep and
        health benefits, 70, 80
    Cauliflower Cranberry Superfood
        Salad, *180*
    Chickpea and Squash Slow Cooker
        Curry, *163*
    Grapefruit Salmon Salad, *164–65*

other recipes with, *174, 175*
    Tropical Chickpea Walnut Quinoa
        Bowl, *154–55*
    Zucchini Ribbons with Chickpeas and
        Olive Oil, *168*
Bedtime snacks, best, 186
Beef, top sirloin steak, 126–27
Berries
    about: history of, 115; how and when
        to enjoy, 114; nutrition facts, 115;
        sleep and health benefits, 114;
        strawberries, 114–15
    Almond Butter Jelly Smoothie, *156*
    Banana and Walnut Trail Mix, *157*
    Berry Coconut Smoothie Bowl, *169*
    Blueberry Cottage Cheese Parfait, *160*
    Cauliflower Cranberry Superfood
        Salad, *180*
Blackened Salmon Tacos, *172–73*
Blood sugar
    insulin sensitivity, diabetes and sleep,
        20–21
    low, impacting sleep, 16
Blueberries. *See* Berries
Bowls. *See* Smoothies and bowls
Bread. *See* Whole-grain bread
Brown rice, 54–55, 163

Caffeine
    amount in various beverages, 33
    coffee and, 28–29
    dark chocolate and, 33–34
    energy drinks and, 30–31
    how to avoid it, 29, 30, 31, 33, 34

Caffeine—*continued*
  recommended consumption limit, *29*
  sodas with, 31–33
  teas and, 30
  timing of consumption, 29
  varying effects of, 28
Calcium
  drinking sodas and, 32
  food sources of, 46, 74, 80, 84, 96–97,
    110, 112, 122, 142
  melatonin production and, 68, 74
  orange juice with, 96–97
  sleep quality and, 16, 68
Cantaloupe, 56–57
Carbohydrates, sleep and, 37–38
Cardiovascular disease, cortisol levels
  and, 20
Carrot Ginger Sauce, *178–79*
Cashews, 58–59
Cauliflower
  about: history of, 61; how and when
    to enjoy, 60–61; nutrition facts, 61;
    sleep and health benefits, 60
  Cauliflower Cranberry Superfood
    Salad, *180*
  Greek Chicken Rice Bowl, *162*
  Sheet Pan Salmon and Vegetables,
    170–71
  Veggie-Stuffed Zucchini, *181*
Celery, 62–63
Cereal, 64–65, *160*. *See also* Grains
Chamomile, 66–67
Checklist for good sleep, 191
Cheese
  about: cottage cheese, 74–75; history
    of, 69; how and when to enjoy, 68;
    nutrition facts, 69; sleep and health
    benefits, 68
  Blueberry Cottage Cheese Parfait, *160*
  Loaded Southwest Sweet Potatoes, *175*
  other recipes with, *151, 153, 162,*
    172–73, 181
  Tofu Patty Melt, *176*
Cherries, tart
  about: history of, 121; how and when
    to enjoy, 120–21; nutrition facts,
    121; sleep and health benefits, 120

  Almond Butter Jelly Smoothie, *156*
  Chocolate Cherry Oatmeal, *150*
  Chocolate Cherry Smoothie, *177*
Chicken rice bowl, Greek, *162*
Chickpeas. *See* Beans and other legumes
Chocolate
  about: dark chocolate, caffeine and
    sleep, 33–34
  Chocolate Banana Oat Bites, *158–59*
  Chocolate Cherry Oatmeal, *150*
  Chocolate Cherry Smoothie, *177*
Citrus
  about: grapefruit, 88–89; history of, 89,
    97; how and when to enjoy, 88–89,
    96; nutrition facts, 89, 97; orange
    juice with calcium, 96–97; sleep and
    health benefits, 88, 96
  Cumin-Lime Dressing, *174*
  Grapefruit Salmon Salad, *164–65*
Coconut water, 72–73
Coffee/caffeine, sleep and, 28–29
Cortisol levels, 16, 19, 20
Cottage cheese, 74–75, *160*
Cucumber
  about: history of, 76–77; how and when
    to enjoy, 76; nutrition facts, 77;
    sleep and health benefits, 76
  Cucumber Tartine, *153*
  other recipes with, *161, 162, 178–79*
Cumin-Lime Dressing, *174*

Dark chocolate, 33–34. *See also*
  Chocolate
Dates, 78–79, *177*
Dehydration, sleep and, 41–42
Diabetes/insulin sensitivity, sleep and,
  20–21
Drinks to avoid for good sleep. *See*
  Caffeine; Foods and drinks to avoid for
  good sleep

Edamame, 80–81, *164–65*
Eggs
  about: history of, 82; how and when to
    enjoy, 82; nutrition facts, 82; sleep
    and health benefits, 82–83
  Egg on Avocado Toast with Salsa, *152*

Greek Quinoa Breakfast Bowl, *151*
Energy drinks, caffeine and sleep, 30–31
Exercise, sleep and, 21–22
Expectations for sleep, 25

Figs, 84–85
Fish
    about: halibut, 90–91; history of, 91,
        109, 111, 129; how and when to
        enjoy, 90–91, 108–9, 110–11, 128–
        29; nutrition facts, 91, 109, 111, 129;
        salmon, 108–9; sardines, 110–11;
        sleep and health benefits, 90, 108,
        110, 128; tuna, 128–29
    Blackened Salmon Tacos, *172–73*
    Grapefruit Salmon Salad, *164–65*
    Sheet Pan Salmon and Vegetables,
        170–71
    Zesty Tuna Lettuce Wraps, *161*
Flaxseed, 86–87
Foods, best for sleep. *See also* Recipes
    about: overview and summary of, 45,
        146
    alphabetic listing of, 46–145. *See also*
        specific foods/ingredients
Foods and drinks to avoid for good sleep,
    27–42. *See also* Caffeine
    about: overview of, 27
    acidic foods, 39–40
    alcohol, 34–36
    best bedtime snacks, 186
    big meals and, 40–41
    dehydration and, 41–42
    refined carbohydrates and sugar,
        37–38
    spicy foods, 39
    three-day meal plan, 182–85
Food/Sleep Log, 187–90
Food-sleep relationship
    about: overview of, 11
    food choices impacting sleep, 16–17
    Food/Sleep Log and, 187–90
    hunger cues and, 17
    low blood sugar and, 16
    overall diet importance, 17
    poor sleep impacting food choices,
        15–16

Goals for sleep, setting, 25
Grains. *See also* Cereal; Quinoa
    about: barley, 52–53; brown rice,
        54–55; history of, 53, 55, 95; how
        and when to enjoy, 52–53, 54–55,
        94–95; nutrition facts, 53, 55, 95;
        oatmeal, 94–95; sleep and health
        benefits, 52, 54, 94
    Chocolate Cherry Oatmeal, *150*
Grapefruit, 88–89, *164–65*
Greek Chicken Rice Bowl, *162*
Greek Quinoa Breakfast Bowl, *151*

Halibut, 90–91
Hunger
    cues, listening to, 17
    hormones, lack of sleep and, 19–20
Hydration, sleep and, 41–42

Insulin sensitivity/diabetes, sleep and,
    20–21

Journaling, sleep and, 23

Loaded Southwest Sweet Potatoes, *175*
Log, for food/sleep, 187–90
Low blood sugar, 16

Magnesium
    alcohol depleting, 35
    benefits and functions, 48, 50, 68, 86,
        88, 90
    food sources of, 46, 48, 50, 58, 68, 70,
        72, 74, 84, 86, 92, 94, 100, 102, 104,
        106, 108, 112, 116, 122, 128, 134,
        142
    importance in chemical reactions in
        body, 104
    for muscle cramps, 68
    serotonin production and, 14
    sleep quality and, 32, 48, 68, 90
Meal plan, three-day, 182–85
Meal size, sleep quality and, 40–41
Meditation, sleep and, 22–23
Melatonin
    antioxidant benefits of, 124
    calcium and production of, 68, 74

Melatonin—*continued*
  food sources of, 45, 46, 76, 100, 120, 124, 134, 150
  functions and characteristics, 14–15
  levels, time of day and, 14–15
  low serotonin levels and, 15
  precursor for production of, 14. *See also* Serotonin
  side effects from supplements, 15
  sleep quality and, 15
  supplements (synthetic), 15
  vitamin B$_6$ importance in production of, 50, 70, 90
Mental health, sleep and, 18
Metabolic disorders and sleep
  cortisol levels, cardiovascular disease and, 20
  hunger hormones and, 19–20
  insulin sensitivity, diabetes and sleep, 20–21
  obesity and, 19
Milk, dairy, 92–93, *150*

Niacin, 14, 47
Nuts
  about: almonds, 46–47; cashews, 58–59; history of, 47, 59, 100–101, 135; how and when to enjoy, 46, 58, 100, 134–35; nutrition facts, 47, 59, 101, 135; pistachios, 100–101; sleep and health benefits, 46, 58, 100, 134; walnuts, 134–35
  Almond Butter Jelly Smoothie, *156*
  Banana and Walnut Trail Mix, *157*
  Chocolate Banana Oat Bites, *158–59*
  Chocolate Cherry Oatmeal, *150*
  Tropical Chickpea Walnut Quinoa Bowl, *154–55*

Oatmeal, 94–95, *150*
Obesity, sleep and, 19
Orange juice with calcium, 96–97

Pasta, whole-grain, 140–41
Peppermint tea, 98–99
Pistachios, 100–101
Portion size, sleep quality and, 40–41

Potassium
  food sources of, 50–51, 60, 62, 68, 70, 72, 74, 76, 78, 80, 84, 88, 92, 96, 102, 112, 114, 118, 124, 136, 142, 144
  functions of, 50, 60
  for muscle cramps, 50
  sleep quality and, 16, 68
  water balance and, 136
Prunes, 102–3
Pumpkin seeds, 104–5, *157*, *164–65*, *180*

Quinoa
  about: history of, 106–7; how and when to enjoy, 106; nutrition facts, 107; sleep and health benefits, 106
  Chickpea and Squash Slow Cooker Curry, *163*
  Greek Quinoa Breakfast Bowl, *151*
  Tropical Chickpea Walnut Quinoa Bowl, *154–55*

Reading before bed, 23–24
Recipes, 150–81
  about: three-day meal plan using, 182–85
  Almond Butter Jelly Smoothie, *156*
  Banana and Walnut Trail Mix, *157*
  Berry Coconut Smoothie Bowl, *169*
  Blackened Salmon Tacos, *172–73*
  Blueberry Cottage Cheese Parfait, *160*
  Cauliflower Cranberry Superfood Salad, *180*
  Chickpea and Squash Slow Cooker Curry, *163*
  Chocolate Banana Oat Bites, *158–59*
  Chocolate Cherry Oatmeal, *150*
  Chocolate Cherry Smoothie, *177*
  Cucumber Tartine, *153*
  Egg on Avocado Toast with Salsa, *152*
  Grapefruit Salmon Salad, *164–65*
  Greek Chicken Rice Bowl, *162*
  Greek Quinoa Breakfast Bowl, *151*
  Loaded Southwest Sweet Potatoes, *175*
  Roasted Summer Vegetable Panzanella, *166–67*

Sheet Pan Salmon and Vegetables, *170–71*
Sweet Potato Fiesta Salad, *174*
Tofu Patty Melt, *176*
Tofu Spring Rolls with Carrot Ginger Sauce, *178–79*
Tropical Chickpea Walnut Quinoa Bowl, *154–55*
Veggie-Stuffed Zucchini, *181*
Zesty Tuna Lettuce Wraps, *161*
Zucchini Ribbons with Chickpeas and Olive Oil, *168*
REM sleep, 12, 13
Rice. *See* Grains
Rice, brown, 54–55, *163*
Roasted Summer Vegetable Panzanella, *166–67*

Salmon. *See* Fish
Sardines, 110–11
Seeds
    about: flaxseed, 86–87; history of, 87, 104–5, 117; how and when to enjoy, 86–87, 104, 116; nutrition facts, 87, 105, 117; pumpkin seeds, 104–5; sleep and health benefits, 86, 104, 116; sunflower seeds, 116–17
    Banana and Walnut Trail Mix, *157*
    Cauliflower Cranberry Superfood Salad, *180*
    Grapefruit Salmon Salad, *164–65*
    Tofu Spring Rolls with Carrot Ginger Sauce, *178–79*
Serotonin
    functions and characteristics, 14
    importance of tryptophan-containing foods for, 14
    low melatonin levels and, 15
    tryptophan connection, 13–14, 15
    vitamin B$_6$ importance in production of, 50, 90
Sleep. *See also* Food-sleep relationship
    bodily repairs during, 12–13
    checklist for good sleep, 191
    deeper stages of, 12–13
    deprivation prevalence, 12
    hours recommended, 12, 25
    lightest stage of, 12
    low blood sugar and, 16
    realistic goals and expectations, 25
    REM, 12, 13
    restorative value of, 12
    stages of, 12–13
Sleep, additional aids for, 21–25. *See also* Foods *references*; Food-sleep relationship; Recipes
    aromatherapy, 24–25
    exercise, 21–22
    general guidelines, 21
    meditation, 22–23
    reading before bed, 23–24
    writing and journaling, 23
Sleep, lack of
    about: overview of impact, 17–18
    food choices causing, 16–17
    impacting food choices, 15–16
    mental health impact, 18
    metabolic disorders and, 19–21
    obesity and, 19
    stress and, 18
Smoothies and bowls
    Almond Butter Jelly Smoothie, *156*
    Berry Coconut Smoothie Bowl, *169*
    Greek Chicken Rice Bowl, *162*
    Tropical Chickpea Walnut Quinoa Bowl, *154–55*
Snacks, best for bedtime, 186
Sodas (caffeinated), sleep and, 31–33
Spicy foods, sleep and, 39
Spinach, 112–13
Squash, *163, 170–71. See also* Zucchini
Stages of sleep, 12–13
Steak, top sirloin, 126–27
Strawberries, 114–15, *169*
Stress
    cortisol levels, cardiovascular disease and, 20
    lack of sleep and, 18
    mental health impact, 18
Sugar, sleep and, 37–38
Sunflower seeds, 116–17, *157, 178–79*
Supplements
    melatonin (synthetic), 15
    tryptophan, 14

Sweet potatoes
about: history of, 119; how and when
to enjoy, 118–19; nutrition facts,
119; sleep and health benefits, 118
Loaded Southwest Sweet Potatoes,
175
Sweet Potato Fiesta Salad, 174

Tacos, blackened salmon, 172–73
Tart cherries. See Cherries, tart
Teas (caffeinated), sleep and, 30
Teas, herbal
chamomile, 66–67
peppermint, 98–99
valerian root, 132–33
Three-day meal plan, 182–85
Tofu
about: history of, 123; how and when
to enjoy, 122–23; nutrition facts,
123; sleep and health benefits, 122
Chocolate Cherry Smoothie, 177
Tofu Patty Melt, 176
Tofu Spring Rolls with Carrot Ginger
Sauce, 178–79
Tomatoes, 124–25, 166–67, 172–73
Top sirloin steak, 126–27
Tropical Chickpea Walnut Quinoa Bowl,
154–55
Tryptophan
food sources of, 13, 82, 86, 90, 106,
110, 128, 130, 134
functions and characteristics, 13–14
importance of eating foods with, 13–14
serotonin connection, 13–14
supplements improving sleep, 14
Tuna, 128–29, 161
Turkey, 130–31

Valerian root tea, 132–33
Veggie-Stuffed Zucchini, 181
Vitamin B$_6$ (pyridoxine)
deficiency effects, 50, 70
food sources of, 51, 52, 56, 70, 78, 90,
94, 100, 102, 108, 110, 116, 118, 126,
128, 130, 136, 138, 140
importance in enzyme reactions, 50
melatonin production and, 50, 70

serotonin production and, 50, 90
sleep quality and, 50
Vitamin D
under consumption of, 16
food sources of, 82, 92, 96, 111

Walnuts, 134–35, 150, 154–55, 157
Water intake, sleep and, 41–42
Watermelon, 136–37
Whole-grain bread
about: history of, 138–39; how and
when to enjoy, 138; nutrition facts,
139; sleep and health benefits, 138
Cucumber Tartine, 153
Egg on Avocado Toast with Salsa, 152
Roasted Summer Vegetable
Panzanella, 166–67
Tofu Patty Melt, 176
Whole-grain pasta, 140–41
Writing, sleep and, 23

Yogurt
about: history of, 143; how and when
to enjoy, 142; nutrition facts, 143;
sleep and health benefits, 142
Almond Butter Jelly Smoothie, 156
Cumin-Lime Dressing, 174

Zesty Tuna Lettuce Wraps, 161
Zucchini
about: history of, 145; how and when
to enjoy, 144–45; nutrition facts,
145; sleep and health benefits, 144
other recipes with, 166–67, 169
Veggie-Stuffed Zucchini, 181
Zucchini Ribbons with Chickpeas and
Olive Oil, 168